DIABETIC
COOKBOOK

Cover design: Jean Provencher

First published in French by
Les Editions La Presse, Montreal, Quebec

Copyright © Gage Educational Publishing Limited 1975
Printed and Bound in Canada

ISBN   0-7715-9926-9 Casebound
        0-7715-9927-7 Paperback

1 2 3 4 5 6 7 8 9   D   80 79 78 77 76 75

Géraldine Thibaudeau
Professional Dietitian

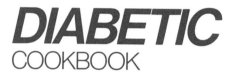

DIABETIC
COOKBOOK

Approved by the
Diabetic Association of Quebec

translated by Marni Jackson

Gage Publishing Limited

Contents

Preface

Diabetics don't always like the idea of dieting, even though this is absolutely fundamental to any treatment of the illness. It's important that they come to accept this, and it's encouraging that there is now a book, reflecting Mlle. Thibaudeau's thorough knowledge of the subject, that will make this task easier.

The author has already broken new ground with the original edition, the first of its kind written in French. From the Diabetic Association of Quebec — and for all diabetics — we offer our warm congratulations. With her help, diabetics will find it easier to enhance their meals without breaking their dietary regulations.

An easier, longer, and more satisfying life — in other words, an almost normal life: this is what Mlle. Thibaudeau offers to all diabetics.

Dr. Rosario Robillard, F.R.C.P.(C)
L.M.C.C.

Introduction

This is a cookbook of special recipes created for diabetics who enjoy good food, despite the serious restrictions imposed on what they may eat.

The aim of this book is to make the task of calculating food exchanges easier. Each recipe carefully lists the permissible ingredients, along with their exact exchange values.

The importance of the family meal, enjoyed together, has also been taken into consideration. "Diabetic" meals are also meals that observe the basic rules of healthy nutrition — a good habit for everyone these days. Your guests can also enjoy the soups, main courses, and desserts presented here, because flavor has not been sacrificed to sound nutrition.

Many of the recipes allow for this flexibility, freeing the cook from the constant chore of preparing a separate menu for the diabetic.

Among the many practical suggestions included are especially useful tips for diabetic children or adults on how to eat sensibly away from home.

In short, these are recipes that you can trust your health with — and they also offer the kind of day-by-day variety in meals that diabetics have been missing.

Foreword

Very simply, this cookbook is intended for the diabetic. In many cases it can be used for other types of diets, and often for the whole family. It offers enough variety to avoid repetition, and at the same time the recipes are easy to prepare. There are countless other tempting recipes that might have been included —someday they may be — but in the meantime, this represents a beginning!

I am indebted to Mme. Michele Tremblay, Director of Diet Therapy at the Sacred Heart Hospital, for a number of recipes which she originated and tested. At every stage of the work, her co-operation has been invaluable. The support and advice of doctors specializing in diabetes have encouraged us to stay with the project, and to share the results of it with you.

It's not as hard as you think to eat well!

Géraldine Thibaudeau

Conversion Tables and Utensils

Table of Equivalent Measures

3 teaspoons	= 1 tablespoon	
2 tablespoons	= 1 oz	= 30 grams
4 tablespoons	= ¼ cup	= 2 oz
8 tablespoons	= ½ cup	= 4 oz
16 tablespoons	= 1 cup	= 8 oz
	1 cup	= 240 cc
2 cups	= 1 pint (U.S.A.)	= 16 oz
2½ cups	= 1 pint (Canada)	= 20 oz
4 cups	= 1 quart (U.S.A.)	= 32 oz
5 cups	= 1 quart (Canada)	= 40 oz
4 quarts (Canada)	= 1 gallon (Canada)	= 160 oz
4 quarts (U.S.A.)	= 1 gallon (U.S.A.)	= 128 oz
15 grams	= 1 tablespoon	
450 grams	= 16 oz	= 1 lb
1000 grams	= 1 kilo	
1 kilo	= 2.2 lbs	
1 gram of proteins	= 4 calories	
1 gram of carbohydrates	= 4 calories	
1 gram of fats	= 9 calories	

Utensils Required for a Prescribed Diet

Set of measuring spoons, for measuring fats and cereals.
Set of four nested cups:

1-cup size — especially convenient for vegetables and milk.
½ cup — for vegetables and fruits.
⅓ cup — useful for some bread exchanges in particular.
¼ cup — handy for cheese, fish, and canned food.

A graduated glass cup for measuring liquids.

Other Useful Equipment

A frying pan reserved for cooking eggs. It should have curved, sloping sides and a Teflon coating to prevent sticking. Don't use this for cooking anything else.
A frying pan with a lid, a saucepan, or a casserole dish, or an enameled roasting pan for braising.
A fairly heavy Teflon frying pan, for cooking meat.
A charcoal hibachi, or preferably a small electric rotisserie.
An assortment of 4- and 6-oz. individual baking dishes, made of fire-proof glass or porcelain; 4-oz. dishes for measured dessert portions.
An assortment of small tart or pudding molds, 3" in diameter, made of light aluminum.
Small set of scales, graduated from 0 to 16 oz.
A blender.
An ice cream scoop, in no. 8 (½ cup) or no. 12 (⅓ cup) size: useful for measuring portions.
Transparent polythene wrapping (for oven-roasting meat and vegetables) either in a roll, or in bags of various sizes.
Saran-Wrap, to cover leftovers.
An assortment of containers with airtight lids, in individual portion sizes, for the freezer.

exchanges

Exchanges

List I — Milk Exchanges

1 exchange of milk contains: carbohydrates: 12 g; fats: 10 g; proteins: 8 g.
Calories: 170. Amount: 8 oz or 240 g.

Whole milk	1 cup or 8 oz or 240 g
Evaporated milk	½ cup or 4 oz or 120 g
Buttermilk	1 cup or 8 oz or 240 g (add two Fat Exchanges)
Skim milk	1 cup or 8 oz or 240 g (add two Fat Exchanges)
Powdered skim milk	¼ cup or 4 tablespoons (add two Fat Exchanges)

List II — Vegetable Exchanges

Group A, or 5%

Eat as much as you like of any of these vegetables that can be eaten raw. The exception is the tomato, which is limited to either a whole one or a half cup of juice per meal. For cooked vegetables, the maximum portion is one cup. Group A nutritional formula: carbohydrates: 3 to 5 g; fats: 0 g; proteins: 2 g.
Calories: less than 30.

Asparagus	Endive
Bean sprouts	Green or yellow beans
Beet leaves	Green Pepper
Broccoli	Lettuce
Brussels sprouts	Mushrooms
Cabbage	Radish
Cauliflower	Sauerkraut
Celery	Spinach
Chard	Summer squash
Chicory	Sweet Pepper
Chinese Cabbage	Tomato or tomato juice
Cucumber	Turnip greens
Dandelion greens	Watercress
Eggplant	

Group B, or 10%

1 exchange (½ cup per serving) contains: carbohydrates: 7 g + or −; fats: 0 g; proteins: 2 g. Calories: about 40.

Beets	Onion
Carrots	Rutabaga
Green peas	Winter squash

Corn (kernel) — limited to ¼ cup.

List III   Fruit Exchanges

Fruit Exchanges are in the 10% category. Raw or cooked, fresh or preserved, tinned or frozen — but unsweetened — the exchange contains: carbohydrates: 10 g; fats: 0 g; proteins: 0 g. Calories: about 40. Amount: variable.

Apple	½ cup, or 1, 2" diameter fruit
Apricots	2 medium, or 4 halves
Banana	Half a small one
Blackberries	1 cup
Blueberries	¾ cup
Cantaloupe	¼ of a 6" diameter fruit
Cherries	10 large
Dates	2
Figs, dried	1 small
Figs, fresh	2 large
Grapes	12 medium
Grape juice	¼ cup or 2 oz
Grapefruit	½ of a 4" diameter fruit
Grapefruit juice	½ cup or 4 oz
Honeydew melon	¾ cup, or ⅛ of an 8" diameter fruit
Ice cream (vanilla, chocolate, strawberry)	⅙ of a pint brick (subtract 1 Fat Exchange)
Mandarins	1 large
Mango	½ a small fruit

Nectarine	1 medium
Orange	1 small
Orange juice	½ cup or 4 oz
Papaya	⅓ of a medium-sized fruit
Peach	1 medium or 2 halves
Pear	1 small or 2 halves
Pineapple	½ cup or 2 slices
Pineapple juice	⅓ cup
Plums	2 medium
Prune juice	¼ cup or 2 oz
Prunes, dried	2 medium
Raisins	2 tablespoons
Raspberries	¾ cup
Strawberries	1 cup
Watermelon	1 cup chopped or 1, 3" x 1½" slice

List IV Bread Exchanges

One bread exchange contains: carbohydrates: 15 g; fats: 0 g; proteins: 2 g; Calories: 68; Amount: about 1 oz or 30 g.

Bread, white or brown	1 regular 1 oz slice
Cereals: cooked	½ cup
raw	¼ cup before cooking
dry — flakes or puffs	¾ cup
Crackers: Graham	4, 2" size
Social tea	4
Saltines	5, 2" size
Soda biscuits	6, 2" size
Ritz	7
Flour, all-purpose	2½ tablespoons
Ice cream	½ cup (subtract two Fat Exchanges)
Melba toast: rectangular	4
round	6

Muffin, plain	1, 2" diameter
Rice, spaghetti, macaroni, vermicelli, etc	½ cup after cooking
Rolls	1, 2" diameter
Sponge cake	1, 1½" cube

Starchy Vegetables

Baked beans (no pork)	¼ cup
Corn: canned	⅓ cup
popcorn (no oil or butter)	1 cup
Parsnip	⅔ cup
Peas and dried beans, cooked	½ cup
Potatoes	1 small
mashed	⅓ cup
Sweet Potato (or Yam)	¼ cup

List V   Meat Exchanges

An exchange of meat contains: carbohydrates: 0 g; fats: 5 g; proteins: 7 g. Calories: 73. Amount: 30 g, or 1 oz.

Bacon, lean and crisp	3 slices
Beef, lamb, liver, pork, poultry, veal	1 oz cooked, and trimmed of fat
Cold cuts: salami, ham, sausage, pressed meat	1 slice, 4½" x ⅛"
Cheese: cheddar	1 oz or 1 commercial slice
grated/hard	4 tablespoons
skim milk	1 oz or 1 commercial slice (add 1 Fat Exchange)
cottage	¼ cup (add 1 Fat Exchange)
Gruyère	1½ wedges
Eggs	1 medium

Eggwhites	2 (add 1 Fat Exchange)
Fish, white	1 oz cooked
Frankfurters (8-9 per lb)	1
Peanut butter	2 tablespoons (limited to one serving per day)
Sardines	3 medium
Sausages, beef (15 - 16 per lb)	1½, cooked and drained
Seafood: salmon, tuna, crab, lobster scallops, oysters,	¼ cup
shrimps	5

List VI Fat Exchanges

One exchange of fat contains: carbohydrates: 0 g; fats: 5 g; proteins: 0 g. Calories: 45. Amount: 1 teaspoon.

Avocado	⅛ of a 4″ diameter fruit
Bacon, crisp	1 slice
Butter or margarine	1 teaspoon or a pat 1″ square x ¼″ thick
Cooking oil or fat	1 teaspoon
Cream: light	2 tablespoons
heavy	1 tablespoon
Cream cheese	1 tablespoon
Mayonnaise, commercial	1 teaspoon
Nuts	6 small
Olives	5 small
Peanuts	10
Salad dressing, commercial	1 tablespoon

The exchanges used here are those used by the American Dietetic Association and the American Diabetes Association. Check your own list of exchanges against these; there may be slight differences, especially in the vegetable groups.

broths and hearty soups

Broths and Hearty Soups

Home-made Soups

If you can count and measure correctly, that's all there is to making soup!

Soup starts with a good stock, always with the fat skimmed off. If home-made stock isn't on hand, the commercial variety can be used. It's available in powder form, crystals, concentrate, or in cubes, and it doesn't contain too much fat.

The easiest approach to begin with is to add ordinary exchanges to whatever amount of stock you want. For example:

—with ⅓ cup cooked rice or noodles, the soup is worth 1 Bread exchange.

—with ½ cup of cooked vegetables (cabbage, beans, tomatoes), the soup is worth 1 Group A (5%) Vegetable Exchange.

—with 1 oz of chopped chicken, the soup is equivalent to 1 Meat Exchange.

—combinations such as noodles and meat, noodles and vegetables, noodles, vegetables, and meat can be tried as well; the soup is always worth the total of the exchanges used.

Cream Soups diluted with water or milk

All the major commercial brands of cream soups have approximately the same value.

Usually, 1 regular size, 10-oz can of soup is diluted with 1 can of water, to make 3 portions, or ⅓ can plus an equal amount of water = 1 portion.

Cream of Green Pea	= **1 Bread Exchange + 1 Fat Exchange**
Cream of Tomato	= **1 Bread Exchange**
Cream of Asparagus	= **½ Bread Exchange + ½ Fat Exchange**
Cream of Celery	= **½ Bread Exchange + 1 Fat Exchange**
Cream of Chicken	= **½ Bread Exchange + 1 Fat Exchange**
Cream of Vegetable	= **½ Bread Exchange + 1 Fat Exchange**

If the same cream soups are diluted with milk, then their real value is increased by the Milk Exchange used.

Soups diluted with water

Commercial soups diluted with water, in the same proportions
(⅓ of a 10-oz can plus ⅓ can of water) have the following values:

Tomato and Rice	= **1 Bread Exchange**
Vegetable	= **1 Bread Exchange**
Beef, Chicken, or Turkey Noodle	= **½ Bread Exchange + ½ Fat Exchange**
Vegetable (no meat stock used)	= **½ Bread Exchange + ½ Fat Exchange**
Chicken and Vegetable	= **½ Meat Exchange + ½ Bread Exchange**
Beef	= **½ Meat Exchange + ½ Bread Exchange**
Beef and Vegetable	= **½ Meat Exchange + ½ Bread Exchange**
Scotch Broth	= **½ Meat Exchange + ½ Bread Exchange**
Clam Chowder	= **½ Meat Exchange + ½ Bread Exchange**
Minestrone	= **½ Bread Exchange + 1 Fat Exchange**

Apple Beef Bouillon

Ingredients	Can of consommé	10 oz
	Apple juice	1 cup
	Cinnamon	1 pinch

Preparation Combine the consommé and apple juice in the saucepan, and bring to a boil.
Serve with a sprinkling of cinnamon.

Portions 3

Exchange Value 1 portion = 1 Group A Vegetable Exchange

Consommé Madrilène

Ingredients	Tomato juice	4 oz
	Apple juice	1 oz

Preparation Mix, heat, and serve immediately.

Portion 1

Exchange Value 1 portion = 1 Group B Vegetable Exchange

Cardinal Consommé

Ingredients	Jellied chicken stock, skimmed	1 cup
	Mixed vegetable juice	½ cup

Preparation Mix and heat.

Portions 2 6-oz portions

Exchange Value The value of a single portion is negligible.

Variation: Garnish with a thin slice of lemon.

Watercress Soup

Ingredients	Chicken stock, skimmed	2½ cups
	Salt	½ teaspoon
	Monosodium glutamate	¼ teaspoon
	Onion, finely chopped	2 tablespoons
	Celery, finely chopped	¼ cup
	Chopped chicken or turkey	1½ cups
	Watercress, finely chopped	1 cup
	Cornmeal	1 tablespoon

Preparation Mix the first six ingredients in a saucepan.
Simmer ten minutes.
Add the watercress and simmer a bit more.
Mix the cornmeal with cold water to make a smooth paste.
Add the paste to the soup, and cook for 5 or 6 minutes, until slightly thickened.

Portions 4

Exchange Value 1 portion = 2 Meat Exchanges + 1 Group A Vegetable Exchange

Parsley Soup

Ingredients	Parsley	1 bunch
	Potatoes, raw, peeled, and diced	6 small
	Lettuce, quartered	1 small head
	Beef or chicken stock	6 cups

Preparation Bring the stock to a boil and add the vegetables.
Season to taste.
Cook over low heat for 30 minutes.
Put the soup in the blender for a smoother texture, and decorate with parsley just before serving.

Portions 6

Exchange Value 1 portion = 1 Bread Exchange

Spinach Soup

Ingredients		
	Fresh spinach, finely chopped	2 cups
	Diced carrots	⅔ cup
	Shallots, finely chopped	6
	Chicken stock	6 cups
	Salt and pepper	to taste

Preparation Add the vegetables to the boiling chicken stock.
Simmer 30 minutes, covered, over a low heat, stirring now and then.

Portions 4

Exchange Value 1 portion = 1 Group A Vegetable Exchange

Corn Soup

Ingredients		
	Corn, finely minced with a vegetable chopper, or put in the blender	⅔ cup
	Cooked rice	⅔ cup
	Chicken stock, defatted	1½ cups
	Skim milk, fresh or reconstituted	1 cup
	Parsley, chopped	2 tablespoons
	Salt	¼ teaspoon
	Thyme	1 pinch

Preparation Gently simmer all the ingredients for five minutes.
Serve immediately.

Portions Divide into 4 portions

Exchange Value 1 portion = 1 Bread Exchange + ¼ Milk Exchange,
or 1 Group A Vegetable Exchange +
1 Group B Vegetable Exchange + ½ Meat Exchange.

Onion Soup

Ingredients

Onions	4 medium
Butter or margarine	4 teaspoons
Beef stock, defatted	3 cups
Salt	½ teaspoon
Pepper	few grains
Celery salt	⅛ teaspoon
Worcestershire sauce	1 teaspoon

Preparation

Slice the onions finely and sauté them until golden in the melted butter or margarine.
Add the stock, and simmer until the onions are cooked.
Season and serve steaming.

Portions   4

Exchange Value

1 portion = 1 Fat Exchange + 1 Group A Vegetable Exchange.

Note

½ cup grated Parmesan cheese, added just before serving, will increase the value by ½ Meat Exchange per portion.

French Onion Soup

Ingredients

Butter	1 tablespoon
Onions, sliced finely	6 medium (size of an egg)
Beef stock	3 cubes
Boiling water	6 cups
Grated Parmesan cheese	2 tablespoons per portion

Preparation

Slowly sauté the sliced onions in the melted butter, until they turn golden.
Use a heavy saucepan that retains the heat well.
Add the reconstituted beef stock, bring to a boil, and simmer for ten minutes.

Sprinkle 2 tablespoons grated Parmesan cheese on each bowl of soup (use ovenproof dishes), and place under the broiler for five minutes.

Portions   6

Variation   Pour the soup into 6 earthenware bowls.
Cover each with a slice of French bread, 4″ × 3″ × ½″.
Sprinkle each with 2 tablespoons grated Parmesan.
Brown under broiler.
In this case, add 1 Bread Exchange to the value.

Exchange Value   1 portion = 1 Group A Vegetable Exchange + ½ Meat Exchange.

Cauliflower Soup

Ingredients		
Cauliflower	1 large
Diced onion	1
Diced carrot	1
Fresh tomatoes, sliced	4
Chopped celery	1 stalk
Chopped parsley	2 tablespoons
Salted boiling water	6 cups
Butter	2 tablespoons

Preparation   Divide the cauliflower into flowerets.
Cook for 25 minutes in the salted boiling water.
Sauté the other vegetables and the parsley in the butter, then add to this half of the water used to cook the cauliflower.
Cook for 30 minutes.
Add the cauliflower, reserving 6 flowerets for decoration.
Purée the soup in the blender, and garnish each portion with parsley and cauliflower.

Portions   6

Exchange Value   1 portion = 1 Group A Vegetable Exchange + 1 Fat Exchange.

Carrot Soup

Ingredients		
	Carrots, peeled and diced	12 medium
	Turnip, peeled and diced	1 small
	Chopped celery	1 stalk
	Butter	1 tablespoon
	Flour	1 tablespoon
	Boiling water	8 cups
	Thyme, salt, pepper, bay leaf	to taste
	Chopped parsley	for garnish

Preparation   Sauté the chopped vegetables in the melted butter.
Sprinkle with the flour, gradually add the boiling water, add the seasonings, and stir steadily to prevent lumps.
Cover and simmer about 40 minutes.
Strain, or use the blender for a smooth texture.
Sprinkle with chopped parsley.

Portions   6

Exchange Value   1 portion = 1 Group B Vegetable Exchange + ½ Fat Exchange.

Quick Vegetable Soup

Ingredients		
	Mixed vegetables, canned or frozen	1 cup
	Beef bouillon	2 cubes
	Boiling water	2 cups
	Seasoning	to taste

Preparation   Dissolve the bouillon cubes in the boiling water.
Crush the vegetables with a fork and add to the stock.
Season to taste, and reheat.

Portions   2, 8-oz portions

Exchange Value   1 portion = 1 Group B Vegetable Exchange.

Green Bean Soup

Ingredients	Beef stock	1 cup
	Puréed green beans	4 oz
	Salt, pepper	to taste

Preparation Heat all the ingredients in a saucepan.
Use a whisk to blend completely.

Exchange Value 1 portion = 1 Group A Vegetable Exchange.

Tomato and Vegetable Soup

Ingredients	Beef stock	2 cubes
	Boiling water	3 cups
	Chicken stock	2 cubes
	Tomato juice	19 oz
	Onion, finely chopped	1
	Shredded carrot	½ cup
	Diced celery	2 stalks
	Whole pepper	3 grains
	Sage	½ teaspoon
	Salt	1 teaspoon

Preparation Assemble all the ingredients in a pot with a tight-fitting lid.
Leave it to simmer over gentle heat for an hour.

Portions 5, 1-cup portions

Exchange Value 1 portion = 1 Group B Vegetable Exchange

Cream of Chicken and Corn

Ingredients	Cooked chicken, diced	¼ cup
	Can of Chicken and Rice Soup, undiluted	10½ oz
	Whole milk	10½ oz
	Creamed corn	8-oz can
	Chopped parsley	2 tablespoons
	Salt	¼ teaspoon
	Thyme	1 pinch

Preparation   Mix the ingredients in a saucepan and simmer covered for five minutes. Serve promptly.

Portions   4

Exchange Value   1 portion = 3 Meat Exchanges + 1 Group A Vegetable Exchange + 1 Group B Vegetable Exchange.

main courses

meat and poultry

Meat and Poultry

Main Courses

For the diabetic, there's always the problem of having to choose a plan for meals, from a limited range of foods, that doesn't become monotonous. Sometimes inspiration can run out. . .

What's on your menu today? The same old thing, cooked apart from everyone else's meal? Then it's time for a new régime!

Let's consider the main course. Every aspect of a meal deserves careful attention, but obviously success hinges, to a large extent, on the main dish.

The choice for the main course can focus on the meat course: pork, beef, lamb, or poultry. And, although they're neglected far too often, don't overlook fish and seafood; they ought to have a regular place in our diet.

Don't forget egg and cheese dishes, either. When they are well prepared, they are full-fledged meals, both appetizing and sustaining.

Swiss Steak

Ingredients		
	½" Steak, shoulder cut, trimmed of fat	1 lb
	Canned tomatoes	16 oz
	Sliced onion	1 medium
	Chopped celery	½ cup
	Salt	¾ teaspoon
	Pepper	⅛ teaspoon
	Marjoram	½ teaspoon
	Garlic powder	¼ teaspoon

Preparation
Season the steak with salt and pepper.
Use meat tenderizer, if desired.
Sear the meat over moderate heat, until both sides are browned.
Add the vegetables and seasonings.
Cover and cook gently for 2½ hours, or until tender.
Check the evaporation of the cooking liquid, and add boiling water if necessary.

Portions
Divide into 4

Exchange Value
1 portion = 3 Meat Exchanges + 1 Group A Vegetable Exchange.

Salt-fried Steak

Ingredients
Beefsteak, reasonably thick
Table salt

Preparation
Divide after cooking for more than one serving.
Use a sturdy frying pan, of cast-iron or aluminum.
Heat until very hot.
Cover the bottom with ¼" of salt and leave it to heat thoroughly.
Place the steak on the bed of hot salt.
Cook 3 or 4 minutes on one side, depending on how well-done you want it.
Turn and cook the other side about 3 minutes.

Note
The steak will turn out perfectly juicy and not too salty.
The preparation also involves no fat.

Cabbage Rolls

Ingredients	Lean veal and beef, chopped	4 oz
	Cooked rice	⅔ cup
	Salt, pepper, onion salt, spices	to taste
	Fresh cabbage leaves	4
	Tomato juice	1 cup
	Lemon juice	1 teaspoon
	Worcestershire sauce	½ teaspoon

Preparation

Blanch the cabbage leaves by plunging them into boiling water for 3 or 4 minutes.

Rinse briefly with cold water, and dry on a tea towel.

Thoroughly mix the meat, rice, and seasonings, and divide into four portions.

Form into "cigars," and wrap each with a cabbage leaf.

Secure with a toothpick or piece of string.

Place in a cast-iron pan or thick aluminum saucepan.

Add the tomato juice and lemon juice, seasoned with the Worcestershire sauce.

Stew gently, covered, for about 1 hour.

Check the cooking liquid to see that it does not completely evaporate, and add a bit of boiling water if necessary.

Portions 2

Exchange Value

2 rolls = 2 Meat Exchanges + 1 Bread Exchange + 1 Group A Vegetable Exchange.

Chop Suey, without bean sprouts

Ingredients	Onion	1 thin slice
	Green pepper, diced	1 ring
	Vegetable oil	1 teaspoon
	Potato, diced	½, small
	Celery, chopped	1 stalk
	Beef bouillon	½ cup
	Cooked beef, cut into cubes	½ cup
	Soya sauce	to taste

Preparation	Brown the onion and the pepper in the hot oil.
	Add the potato and celery.
	Add the bouillon.
	Cook very gently, covered, for 3 to 5 minutes.
	Add the meat and soya sauce.
	Season with salt and pepper, to taste.
	Reheat before serving.
Exchange Value	1 portion = 2 Meat Exchanges + 1 Group A Vegetable Exchange + 1 Fat Exchange.

Curried Chicken Salad

Ingredients		
	Pre-cooked rice	¾ cup
	Cooked carrots, sliced round	¼ cup
	Special French Sauce (see chapter on sauces)	¼ cup
	Special Salad dressing (see chapter on sauces)	¼ cup
	Black pepper	to taste
	Salt	¾ teaspoon
	Curry powder	¾ teaspoon
	Milk	2 tablespoons
	Cooked chicken or turkey, cut into cubes	2 cups
	Green pepper or lettuce, chopped	¼ cup
	Red onion, chopped or grated	1 small

Preparation Add carrots to the pre-cooked rice and mix with the French Sauce. Cover and refrigerate.

Add the salt, pepper, and curry powder to the Special Salad Dressing, beat thoroughly, and add the milk.

Combine the green pepper, onion, and chicken in a bowl, and pour the curry mixture over it.

Cover and refrigerate for at least 2 hours.

Combine both mixtures just before serving.

Portions Divide into 4 servings and arrange on lettuce leaves.

Exchange Value 1 portion = 2 Meat Exchanges + 1 Bread Exchange + 1 Fat Exchange.

Italian Chicken Marengo

Ingredients

A frying chicken, cut into pieces	3 lbs
Salt and pepper	to taste
Vegetable oil	4 teaspoons
Canned tomatoes	1 cup
Green pepper, sliced, with seeds removed	1 medium
Sliced onions	2 medium
Minced garlic	1 clove
Sliced mushrooms	1 cup

Preparation

Salt and pepper the pieces of chicken.
Heat the oil over a moderate heat in a saucepan or frying pan.
Brown the chicken on all sides until golden.
Add the tomatoes, green pepper, onion, and garlic.
Add more salt and pepper if needed.
Cook covered, over gentle heat, for 40 minutes.
Add the mushrooms.
Continue to cook gently for about 20 minutes, or until the chicken is tender.
Divide into 4 portions.

Exchange Value

1 portion = 3 Meat Exchanges + 1 Group A Vegetable Exchange + 1 Fat Exchange.

Braised Beef and Vegetables

Ingredients

Lean beef, shoulder cut, in 1½" cubes	1 lb
Flour	1 tablespoon
Margarine	4 teaspoons
Chopped onion	¼ cup
Tomato juice	19 oz
Chopped celery	½ cup
Salt	½ teaspoon
Pepper	⅛ teaspoon
Bay leaf	1
Cloves	6 whole

Carrots, sliced round	**2 medium**
Frozen peas	**10 oz**
Chopped green pepper, with seeds removed	**1 medium**

Preparation   Roll the cubes of meat in the flour.
Melt the margarine in a heavy pot.
Brown the meat, then add the chopped onion, and cook until golden.
Add the tomato juice, and scrape the bottom of the pot to incorporate any crust that may have formed.
Add the celery and seasonings, and bring to a boil.
Lower the heat and cover; stew gently for 1½ hours.
Add the carrots and continue to cook for 15 minutes.
Add the peas and green pepper, cook 5 to 10 minutes longer, or until all the ingredients are tender.

Portions   Divide into 4 portions.

Exchange Value   1 portion = 3 Meat Exchanges + 1 Fat Exchange + 1 Group A Vegetable Exchange + 1 Group B Vegetable Exchange.

Baked Chicken and Noodle

Ingredients
Cooked noodles	**⅓ cup**
Cooked chicken, cut into small pieces	**½ cup or 2 oz**
Chicken bouillon	**¼ cup**
Butter	**1 teaspoon**
Mushrooms and green pepper	**to taste**

Preparation   Mix the ingredients in a bowl, place in a ramekin or small baking dish, and bake in a moderate (325 degrees F) oven.

Exchange Value   1 ramekin = 1 Bread Exchange + 2 Meat Exchanges + 1 Fat Exchange.

Note   Several ramekins can be prepared at the same time and frozen.

Stuffed Pork Chops

Ingredients		
8 lean pork chops, very thinly sliced flattened into cutlets	1 lb	
Chopped onion	1	
Chopped celery	2 tablespoons	
Chopped parsley	2 tablespoons	
Butter	8 teaspoons	
Salt	½ teaspoon	
Poultry seasoning	½ teaspoon	
Pepper	to taste	
Fresh bread crumbs	2 cups	
Chicken bouillon, defatted	½ cup	
Flour	2 tablespoons	

Preparation

Lightly pound the cutlets to make them into thin fillets.

Melt half the butter, and sauté the onion, parsley, and celery over gentle heat.

Add the seasonings.

Remove from the heat, and place in a bowl.

Add the breadcrumbs, dampened with a bit of water, and mix gently.

Divide into 8 equal portions and place each on a pork fillet.

Roll and secure with a skewer, or tie with string.

Dredge in flour sprinkled on waxed paper.

Brown in a frying pan, using the rest of the butter.

Add the chicken stock, lower the heat, cover and cook very slowly—about 1½ hours.

Exchange Value

2 chops = 3 Meat Exchanges + 1 Bread Exchange + 2 Fat Exchanges.

Individual Meat Pies

Ingredients

Special pie crust (see the recipe in the chapter on Starchy Foods)	
Lean beef and veal, chopped	1 lb
Cinnamon, nutmeg, cloves	pinch
Dried onion, salt, pepper	optional

44

Preparation	Preheat the oven to 400 degrees.
	Roll the piecrust dough very thin, and cut 8, 4"-diameter circles.
	Brown the meat with the seasonings over low heat.
	Drain off the fat, and divide into 4 equal portions.
	Line 4 small aluminum pie plates (3" diameter) with the pastry circles.
	Fill with the meat.
	Cover each with a round of pastry.
	Score the edges with a fork, and prick the surface.
	Bake for 10 minutes, or until the crust is well browned.
Portions	4 small pies
Exchange Value	1 small pie = 2 Bread Exchanges + 3 Fat Exchanges + 3 Meat Exchanges.

Chicken Livers and Bacon

Ingredients	**Lean bacon**	**4 slices**
	Chopped onion	**1 medium**
	Chicken livers	**1 lb**
	Salt and pepper	**to taste**

Preparation	Fry the bacon slowly, and drain on paper towels.
	Using only 4 teaspoons of the fat left in the frying pan, sauté the onions for 3 minutes, until golden.
	Add the chicken livers, and sauté, turning them frequently with a spatula.
	Cover and cook gently for 10 minutes, stirring occasionally.
	Add salt and pepper.
Portions	Divide into 8 portions, each accompanied by half a slice of bacon.
Exchange Value	1 portion = 2 Meat Exchanges + 1 Fat Exchange.

Broiled Flank Steak

Ingredients		
	Flank steak	2 lbs
	Salt	optional
	Italian salad dressing (low-calorie)	½ cup
	Garlic (pressed)	1 clove
	Prepared mustard	½ teaspoon
	Oregano	¼ teaspoon
	Tabasco sauce	⅛ teaspoon

Preparation
Preheat the broiler.
Mix together the salad dressing, garlic, and spices.
Salt the steak lightly, if desired.
Place on the rack of a broiling pan, and broil 4″ from the element, for 5 to 8 minutes each side (more if you like your steak well done), basting it often with the sauce.

Portions
Divide into 8 equal portions.

Exchange Value
1 portion = 3 Meat Exchanges.

Note
Use a well-sharpened knife and slice the steak diagonally, to obtain 8 thin portions.

Beef and Onion Stew

Ingredients		
	Round steak, cut into 1″ cubes	1½ lbs
	Butter or margarine	2 tablespoons
	Onions	6 medium
	Hot water	3 tablespoons
	Bay leaf	1
	Diced carrots	2½ cups
	French-style green beans (cut lengthwise) thawed and drained	1½ cups
	Salt and pepper	to taste

Preparation	Brown the meat in the butter or margarine, over medium heat. Add 2 finely chopped onions. Add hot water and the bay leaf. Cover and simmer gently for 1½ hours. Check the rate of evaporation; add hot water if necessary. Quarter the rest of the onions, and add them along with the carrots, beans, and spices. Continue cooking in a 350-degree oven, until the vegetables are tender.
Portions	Divide into 6 portions
Exchange Value	1 portion = 3 Meat Exchanges + 1 Bread Exchange + 1 Fat Exchange.

Braised Beef Liver with Mushrooms

Ingredients		
	Margarine	4 teaspoons
	4 slices of liver, of equal thickness	1 lb
	Chopped onion	¼ cup
	Canned mushrooms, juice included	4 oz
	Chopped parsley	1 tablespoon
	Lemon juice	1 tablespoon
	Salt	½ teaspoon
	Pepper	⅛ teaspoon

Preparation	Heat the margarine, and brown both sides of the liver over moderate heat. Add the other ingredients. Simmer covered over low heat for about 10 minutes, or until tender.
Portions	Divide equally among 4 guests.
Exchange Value	1 portion = 3 Meat Exchanges + 1 Fat Exchange + 1 Group A Vegetable Exchange.

Stuffed Ham

Ingredients		
	2 half-inch slices of ham, with the fat trimmed off	total: 1½ lbs
	Whole cloves	12
	Shallots, or onions, finely chopped	4 or 5
	Fresh or frozen spinach	¼ lb
	Chopped celery leaves	½ cup
	Chopped parsley	
	Salt	1 teaspoon
	Pepper	⅛ teaspoon
	Cayenne, nutmeg	1 pinch

Preparation Stud the slices of ham with 6 cloves each.
Combine all the ingredients, and place on one slice of ham.
Lay the other slice on top, and secure with a skewer.
Place on a broiling pan, and bake in a 325-degree oven for about 1½ hours.

Portions Divide into 6 equal portions

Exchange Value 1 portion = 3 Meat Exchanges.
Or: 2 Meat Exchanges, if the ham is divided into 8 portions.

Frankfurter Hash

Ingredients		
	Boiled potatoes, diced and cooled	2⅓ cups
	Chopped onion	1 medium
	Salt and pepper	to taste
	Flour	2 tablespoons
	Milk	¼ cup
	Hot dogs, cut in thin slices	8
	Butter or margarine	4 teaspoons
	Grated cheddar cheese (mild or strong)	½ cup

Preparation	Mix the potatoes and onions in an ovenproof dish.
	Sprinkle with flour, and season with salt and pepper.
	Add the milk and mix in well.
	Cover with the frankfurter slices, and dot with butter.
	Bake in a hot oven (425 degrees) for 30 minutes.
	Sprinkle with grated cheese, and heat five minutes more, or until the cheese forms a crust.
Portions	Divide into 4 equal portions.
Exchange Value	1 portion = 3 Meat Exchanges + 1 Fat Exchange + 2 Bread Exchanges.

Cornish Hen

Ingredients	**Grouse, or Rock Cornish Hen**	**1 lb bird**
	Lemon	**1 quarter**
	Salt and pepper	**to taste**

Preparation	The day before preparation, thaw the "hen" (actually a game bird, not a chicken) in the refrigerator.
	Several hours before cooking, briskly rub the bird inside and out with the lemon section.
	Return to the refrigerator.
	Preheat the oven to 425 degrees.
	Place the bird in a transparent roasting bag, add salt and pepper, and seal.
	Cook 20 minutes in a small roasting pan.
	Lower the heat to 350°F.
	Continue cooking for at least 40 minutes, turning the bird once so that it browns evenly.
Portions	2, 3-oz portions
Exchange Value	1 portion = 3 Meat Exchanges.

Lamb Cutlets with green beans

Ingredients	Margarine	4 teaspoons
	Lean lamb chops, 1″ thick	4
	Chopped onion	¼ cup
	Vegetable stock	1 cube
	Boiling water	¾ cup
	Salt	½ teaspoon
	Pepper	⅛ teaspoon
	Basil	¼ teaspoon
	Frozen French-style green beans (sliced lengthwise)	19 oz

Preparation   Melt the margarine in a saucepan, and brown the chops on both sides.
Remove them from the pan and sauté the onions until golden.
Before returning the chops to the pan, pour off the excess fat.
Add the reconstituted stock, and season with salt, pepper, and basil.
Cover and simmer gently for 15 minutes.
Add the beans, and continue cooking for 5 to 10 minutes, or until tender.

Portions   Divide the chops and vegetables among 4 guests.

Exchange Value   1 portion = 3 Meat Exchanges + 1 Fat Exchange
+ 1 Group A Vegetable Exchange.

Meatballs in tomato sauce

Ingredients	Dried onion flakes	1 tablespoon
	Warm water	1 tablespoon
	Lean beef, minced	1 lb
	Minced garlic	1 clove
	Chopped parsley	1 tablespoon
	Lightly beaten egg	1
	Salt	¼ teaspoon
	Vegetable oil	4 teaspoons

Preparation   Moisten the onion flakes in a bowl with the warm water.
Add the meat, garlic, parsley, egg, and salt, and mix well.
Press firmly into 12 balls.
Heat the oil in a Teflon frying pan, over moderate heat.
Brown the meatballs evenly, and add to the special Tomato Sauce
(see the recipe in the chapter on sauces).

**Exchange
Value**   3 Meatballs = 3 Meat Exchanges + 1 Fat Exchange.

Chicken Chop Suey

Ingredients		
1 roasting chicken	**2 lb bird**	
Chopped green pepper	**½ cup**	
Chopped celery	**1 cup**	
Chopped onion	**½ cup**	
Bean sprouts	**2 cups**	
Flour	**2 tablespoons**	
Soya sauce	**2 tablespoons**	
Canned mushrooms (small pieces)	**½ cup**	
Salt and pepper	**to taste**	

Preparation   Stew the chicken until tender in a well-seasoned stock; it should
be easy to bone, but not overcooked.
Pour off the stock.
Cut the chicken meat into small pieces.
Cook the celery, onion, and pepper slowly in 1 cup of the stock.
Add the chicken and bean sprouts.
Add the flour to the rest of the stock, blend it in, and continue
cooking a few minutes until the flour is completely cooked.
Pour the sauce on the chicken, and add the soya sauce and
mushrooms.

Portions   Divide into 4 equal portions

**Exchange
Value**   1 portion = 3 Meat Exchanges + 1 Group B Vegetable Exchange.

Vegetable Meatloaf

Ingredients		
Green pepper, with seeds removed	1
Peeled carrots	2
Peeled potatoes	2
Peeled onions	2
Chopped lean beef	2 lbs
Lightly beaten eggs	2
Tomato juice	1½ cups
Dry breadcrumbs	½ cup
Salt	1½ teaspoons
Pepper	to taste

Preparation

Chop the vegetables finely with a vegetable chopper.
Mix together all the ingredients.
Press into a bread pan (9″ × 5″ × 3″), or in a square oven glass dish.
Bake in a moderate oven (325 degrees) for about 1½ hours.
Cool for 10 minutes before turning out of the pan.
Serve warm or cold.

Portions

Divide into 9 equal portions

Exchange Value

1 portion = 3 Meat Exchanges + 1 Group B Vegetable Exchange
+ 1 Group A Vegetable Exchange.
However, if the dish is divided into 18 portions, the Exchange value is
1 portion = 2 Meat Exchanges + 1 Group B Vegetable Exchange.

Beef Croquettes

Ingredients		
Stale bread, diced	3 slices
Minced onion	⅓ cup
Green pepper, finely chopped	2 tablespoons
Salt	1 teaspoon
Catsup	¼ cup
Lean beef, chopped	1 lb
Egg	1 whole
Horseradish	1 tablespoon
Dry mustard	½ teaspoon

Preparation	Before measuring the ingredients, preheat the oven to 400 degrees.
	Thoroughly mix all the ingredients in a bowl.
	Divide into 4 equal portions, and shape into croquettes.
	Place on a baking sheet, and bake in the oven for 15 to 20 minutes.

Portions 4

**Exchange
Value** 1 portion = 3 Meat Exchanges + 1 Bread Exchange.

Minced Lamb

Ingredients	**Fresh lamb, minced or finely ground**	**1½ lbs**
	Stale breadcrumbs	**¾ cup**
	Chopped onion	**1**
	Milk	**1½ cups**
	Salt	**2 teaspoons**
	Pepper	**to taste**
	Vegetable oil	**2 tablespoons**

Preparation Mix together all the ingredients, except the oil.
Shape the mixture into 12 small balls; rinsing the hands with cold water makes this easier.
Heat the oil in a thick frying pan (enameled iron, aluminum, or Teflon).
Brown the meatballs.
Cover, lower the heat and continue cooking slowly.
Accompany with special curry sauce (see chapter on sauces).

Portions 12 meatballs

**Exchange
Value** 2 meatballs = 3 Meat Exchanges + 1 Fat Exchange
                      + 1 Group A Vegetable Exchange.
1 meatball = 2 Meat Exchanges.

Note The cooking can be done at the table, in an electric frying pan or in a fondu pot placed over an alcohol flame.

Chicken Liver Pâté

Ingredients		
	Butter	⅛ lb
	Chicken livers	1 lb
	Minced shallots	2
	Salt	1 teaspoon
	Nutmeg	1 pinch
	Pepper, freshly ground	to taste

Preparation

Gently sauté the livers in the butter for 8 to 10 minutes, turning them often with a spatula or wooden spoon so that they cook uniformly.

Reduce the livers to a smooth paste, while adding the seasonings, in a meat grinder or blender.

Press into a glass pan—square or rectangular, to simplify dividing it into equal portions.

Refrigerate 24 hours before serving.

Portions 12

Exchange Value

1 portion = 1 Meat Exchange + 1 Fat Exchange.

Note

You can freeze the pâté in 12 small plastic molds, so that individual portions are always on hand.

Spread on toast; this is a good breakfast substitute for butter and an egg.

It can also be used as a sandwich filling.

Chicken in mushroom sauce

Ingredients		
	Canned cream of mushroom soup	¾ cup
	Chicken stock, defatted and strained	½ cup
	Celery, finely chopped	1 teaspoon
	Chopped green pepper	half a pepper
	Parsley, finely chopped	1 teaspoon
	Cooked chicken, diced	1½ cups
	Toast	4 slices

Preparation	Dilute the cream of mushroom with the half cup of stock.
	Add the celery, green pepper, and parsley.
	Bring to a boil, immediately lower the heat, and stir with a whisk while it simmers.
	Continue to simmer a while, add the chicken, and heat a few more minutes.
Portions	Divide into 4 equal parts. Pour the sauce on 4 slices of toast.
Exchange Value	1 portion = 1 Bread Exchange + 1 Group A Vegetable Exchange + 2 Meat Exchanges + 1 Fat Exchange.

Stuffed Viennese Sausage

Ingredients		
	Unsweetened relish	¼ cup
	Chili sauce	¼ cup
	Prepared mustard	2 teaspoons
	Dried onion flakes	2 teaspoons
	1-oz cheese slices, cut in small pieces	4 slices
	Frankfurters or hot dogs	8
	Hot rolls	8

Preparation	Mix the condiments.
	Add the onion and cheese to make the stuffing.
	Split the frankfurters lengthwise, without cutting them in half.
	Fill each frankfurter with an equal amount of stuffing.
	Place on a baking sheet, and heat in the oven, or broil for about 5 minutes, not too close to the element.
	Serve in the rolls which have been wrapped in aluminum foil and warmed in the oven.
Portions	8
Exchange Value	1 portion = 2 Bread Exchanges + 2½ Meat Exchanges.

main courses

fish and seafood

Fish and Seafood

Tuna Casserole au Gratin

Ingredients	Elbow macaroni	raw: 1 cup or cooked: 2 cups
	Butter or margarine	4 teaspoons
	Chopped onion	¼ cup
	Flour	¼ cup
	Salt	½ teaspoon
	Pepper	⅛ teaspoon
	Dry mustard	1 teaspoon
	Skim milk, fresh or reconstituted	2 cups
	Canned tuna, drained and flaked with a fork	2, 7-oz cans
	Cooked carrots, diced	1 cup
	Grated cheddar cheese	½ cup

Preparation Cook the macaroni in well-salted water for 8 or 9 minutes. Drain immediately.

Or: rinse with cold water after 4 or 5 minutes of cooking, to remove some of the starch. Return to a boil and continue cooking.

Preheat the oven to 375°.

Sauté the onions until golden in the melted butter.

Sprinkle with the flour, and blend in well with a wooden spoon.

Add the salt, pepper, and mustard.

Gradually pour in the room-temperature milk, stirring until it thickens.

Add the macaroni, tuna, and carrots, and slowly bring to the boiling point.

Turn into a glass casserole or fireproof porcelain dish (5-cup capacity).

Sprinkle with the grated cheese, and bake in the oven until the crust is crisp, for 20 minutes.

Portions Divide into 8 equal portions.

Exchange Value 1 portion = 1 Bread Exchange + 2 Meat Exchanges
+ ½ Fat Exchange + ¼ Milk Exchange.
2 portions = 2 Bread Exchanges + 4 Meat Exchanges
+ 1 Fat Exchange + ½ Milk Exchange
+ 1 Group A Vegetable Exchange.

White Fish in Tomato Sauce

Ingredients		
	Fish fillets	1 lb
	Chopped onion	⅔ cup
	Butter or margarine	2 teaspoons
	Flour	2 teaspoons
	Bouillon	1 cube
	Boiling water	½ cup
	Catsup	4 tablespoons
	Dill pickles, sliced	¼ cup

Preparation
Preheat the oven to 450 degrees.
Place the fish in a very lightly greased baking dish.
Sauté the onions until golden in the butter or margarine.
Sprinkle with the flour, and blend with a wooden spoon.
Gradually add the stock.
Add the catsup and simmer 10 minutes, until small bubbles appear, but not beyond the boiling point.
Stir often to prevent lumps.
Add the slices of pickle, and pour over the fish.
Bake for 15 minutes.

Portions
Divide into 4 portions.

Exchange Value
1 portion = 3 Meat Exchanges + 1 Group A Vegetable Exchange + 1 Fat Exchange.

Baked Salmon and Celery

Ingredients		
	Canned salmon, flaked with a fork	1 cup
	Canned cream of celery soup	¾ cup
	Salt, pepper	to taste

Preparation
Mix the ingredients together.
Divide equally between 4 individual ramekins or baking dishes.
Bake in a moderate oven (325°) until the top is crisp and brown.

Exchange Value
1 portion = 1 Meat Exchange + 1 Group A Vegetable Exchange.

Crab Salad

Ingredients		
Fresh, canned, or frozen asparagus		18 spears
Zero Salad Dressing (see the recipe in the chapter on sauces)		1 tablespoon
Lemon juice		1 tablespoon
Zero Mayonnaise (see chapter on sauces)		3 tablespoons
Horseradish		½ teaspoon
Dried onion flakes		¾ teaspoon
Chopped celery		½ cup
Canned crab, drained and flaked		7½ oz
Lettuce leaves		6 large
Hard-boiled eggs, cut in half		3
Olives		15
Medium-sized cucumber		¾
Shallots		3
Tomato slices		6

Preparation

Sprinkle the asparagus with the salad dressing.

Beat together the lemon juice, mayonnaise, horseradish, and onion.

Carefully mix in the celery and crab.

Chill all the ingredients (below) in the refrigerator for an hour.

Arrange them on 3 plates in the following individual proportions: 2 lettuce leaves to cover the plate; 6 asparagus spears, ½ cup of crab, 2 egg halves, 5 olives, a quarter of the cucumber, sliced lengthwise, 1 shallot, and 2 tomato slices.

Decorate with a sprig of watercress, if desired.

Portions

3

Exchange Value

1 portion = 3 Meat Exchanges + 1 Fat Exchange + 1 Group B Vegetable Exchange.

Crab Thermidor

Ingredients		
	White sandwich bread	4 thin slices
	Butter or margarine	4 teaspoons
	Flour	1 tablespoon
	Evaporated Milk	½ cup
	Salt	½ teaspoon
	Nutmeg	⅛ teaspoon
	Paprika, pepper, garlic salt	to taste
	Water	2 tablespoons
	Frozen or canned crab	12 oz
	Cheddar cheese	2 oz

Preparation

Preheat the oven to 350 degrees.
Toast the bread.
In a saucepan, blend the flour into the melted butter with a wooden spoon.
Gradually add the milk, stirring constantly until the sauce thickens.
Season and add the water and the crab, which has been thawed, drained, and flaked with a fork.
Bring to a boil while stirring gently.
Pour in a baking dish, sprinkle with grated cheese.
Broil in the oven until a golden crust is formed.

Portions

Divide into 4 portions.
Pour the sauce on the slices of toast, whole or cut in two.

Exchange Value

1 portion = 1 Bread Exchange + 1 Fat Exchange + ¼ Milk Exchange + 3 Meat Exchanges.

Shrimp Cocktail

Ingredients		
	One lettuce leaf	fresh
	Shrimps	5
	Chili sauce	1 tablespoon
	Horseradish	1 tablespoon
	Lemon	1 slice

Preparation	Line the bottom of a dessert cup or cocktail glass with a lettuce leaf.
	Place the shrimps on it, and top with the horseradish and chili sauce mixture.
	To sharpen the taste, add a lemon slice, squeezing a bit of the juice over the cocktail. Serve very cool.
Portion	One
Exchange Value	1 portion = 1 Meat Exchange.
Note	This cocktail is often served with Oyster biscuits; 10 of these = ½ a Bread Exchange.

Halibut Royale

Ingredients	Halibut steak	1 lb
	Juice of 1 lemon	
	Salt	½ teaspoon
	Paprika, cayenne pepper	¼ teaspoon
	Chopped onion	¼ cup
	Butter or margarine	4 teaspoons
	Green pepper, cut in strips	to garnish

Preparation	Place the fish on a lightly greased baking dish.
	Sprinkle with lemon juice and the seasonings.
	Marinate for an hour in the refrigerator, turning the fish once.
	Preheat the oven to 450° in the meantime.
	Sauté the onion in the butter, and pour over the fish. Garnish with pepper strips, and bake in the oven for 10 minutes.
Portions	Divide into 4 equal portions
Exchange Value	1 portion = 3 Meat Exchanges + 1 Group A Vegetable Exchange + 1 Fat Exchange.

Tomatoes Stuffed with Salmon

Ingredients		
	Tomatoes	6 medium
	Canned salmon, drained and flaked	16 oz
	Chopped celery	½ cup
	Green pepper, finely chopped	¼ cup
	Minced onion	1 tablespoon
	Sesame seeds	1 tablespoon
	Salt	to taste
	Dried mustard	⅛ teaspoon
	Pepper	1 pinch
	Lemon juice	2 tablespoons
	Zero Mayonnaise (see chapter on sauces)	3 tablespoons
	Hard-boiled eggs	2

Preparation Slice off the top of each tomato, and hollow out the inside with a spoon. Drain by turning upside-down on a plate.
Mix together the ten stuffing ingredients.
Cut the eggs in half and carefully remove the yolks.
Crumble one of the yolks, and blend into the stuffing.
Fill each tomato with a sixth of the amount.
Garnish with the other crumbled yolk.

Portions 6

Exchange Value 1 portion = 3 Meat Exchanges + 1 Group A Vegetable Exchange.

Stuffed Halibut

Ingredients		
	2 or more fillets of halibut	1 lb
	Pressed garlic	to taste
	Margarine	4 teaspoons
	Minced onion	½ cup
	Lemon juice	2 teaspoons
	Curry powder	⅛ teaspoon
	Tabasco sauce	⅛ teaspoon
	Tomato slices	4 small

Preparation	Preheat the oven to 350 degrees.
	Press the garlic clove(s) over the fish, and let the fillets absorb it for a while.
	Gently sauté the onions until golden, in the melted margarine.
	Add the lemon juice, curry, and tabasco sauce.
	Cook for 3 minutes.
	Place 1 fillet on a lightly greased baking dish; cover with 4 tomato slices, side by side.
	Remove the onion from the frying pan with a slotted spatula, and spread the drained onions over the tomatoes.
	Place the other fillet on top, and baste with the seasoned cooking liquid.
	Bake in the oven for 30 minutes, or until the fish can be flaked with a fork.
	Decorate with fresh parsley if desired.
Portions	Divide into 4 portions
Exchange Value	1 portion = 3 Meat Exchanges + 1 Fat Exchange + 1 Group A Vegetable Exchange.

Fish Chowder

Ingredients		
	Diced celery	**4 stalks**
	Diced green pepper	**2 medium**
	Shredded cabbage	**2 cups**
	Dried onion flakes	**1 tablespoon**
	Chickel bouillon	**2 cubes**
	Boiling water	**1 cup**
	Tomato juice	**1 19-oz can**
	Thyme	**½ teaspoon**
	Packaged frozen fillets of haddock (cut into 1½" × 2" pieces)	**1 lb**

Preparation	Combine all the ingredients in a saucepan.
	Cover and simmer gently for 10 minutes.
	For a thicker chowder, reduce by continuing to cook, uncovered, for 5 minutes.

Portions   Divide into 4 equal portions

**Exchange
Value**   1 portion = 3 Meat Exchanges + 1 Group A Vegetable Exchange.

Stuffed Fish Fillets

Ingredients		
	Frozen packaged fish fillets	1 lb
	Vegetable or chicken stock	1 package or 1 cube
	Boiling water	½ cup
	Chopped carrot	½ cup
	Chopped celery	¼ cup
	Salt and pepper	to taste
	Flour	3 tablespoons
	Milk	¾ cup
	Marjoram	⅛ teaspoon
	Chopped parsley	1 tablespoon

Preparation Thaw the fish and separate into 4 fillets.
In a saucepan, dissolve the package of stock or bouillon cube in
the boiling water.
Add the carrot and celery, and simmer, covered, for 10 minutes.
Strain and reserve the broth for the sauce.
Place 2 tablespoons of the vegetables near the end of each fillet;
roll and secure with a toothpick.
Return the broth to the saucepan.
Using a whisk or wooden spoon, blend in the flour; gradually pour
in the milk, add the parsley and marjoram, and bring to a boil.
Lower the heat and add the stuffed fillets.
Cover and simmer gently for 15 minutes or less, until the fish
is done.
Accompany each serving with 2 tablespoons of sauce.

Portions   4

**Exchange
Value**   1 portion = 3 Meat Exchanges + ½ Bread Exchange.

main courses

eggs and cheese

Eggs and Cheese

Eggs and Cheese

It's superbly easy to dress up an omelette, and we have listed a few of the possible variations below. Remember that in every one of these recipes, water is a perfectly good substitute for milk. Omelettes are simple to prepare, either in the oven, or in one of the new frying pans coated with an anti-adhesive surface, to keep food from sticking. This means you can save your allotment of butter for another use.

If you feel like having a 2- or 3-egg omelette, you can substitute eggs for your regular portion of meat, according to the specifications of your own diet.

Vary Your Omelette With:

— Herbs
— Vegetables (asparagus, peas, onions, tomatoes, mushrooms, cooked celery).
— Cheese (replace 1 egg with 1 oz of skim milk cheese).
— Fish (replace 1 egg with 1 oz of cooked or canned fish).
— Souffléd Omelette: For a fluffy omelette, separate the whites from the yolks; beat the egg whites stiff, and fold them into the beaten egg yolks, along with the seasonings.
— Stuffed Omelette: Place vegetables in the middle and fold over.
— Ham or Bacon Omelette: Use either 2 eggs and 1 oz of crisp, well-drained bacon, or 2 eggs and 1 oz of lean, chopped ham.
Note: Make allowances for the requirements of your personal diet.

Other Ways to Prepare Eggs

Devilled eggs, or stuffed eggs for salads: Simply blend the yolk of a hard-boiled egg with different seasonings and refill the whites with it.
Baked eggs: Break an egg in a pyrex dish containing 1 teaspoon of milk and seasonings. Top the egg with your allotment of butter or 1 portion of grated cheese, and cook gently in a slow oven (325°).

Baked eggs and spinach: Prepare the same as above, only prepare a bed of well-drained and seasoned spinach in the bottom of the dish. Break the egg(s) into it. The dish can be topped with a portion of butter, or a portion of grated cheese. (Value: 1 Group A Vegetable Exchange + 1 or 2 Meat Exchange + 1 Fat Exchange)

Baked eggs on toast: Lightly butter a slice of fresh bread (crusts removed) and arrange it as a nest in a muffin pan. Let the bread dry in the oven, then break an egg onto the bread. Season and cover with the rest of the butter portion. Bake gently in a **slow** oven, until the bread is golden, and the egg is well done.

Scrambled eggs: Prepare as you would an omelette, and simply cook in a double boiler or a frying pan, without fat, stirring constantly. Cook them soft. All the omelette variations can be done with scrambled eggs.

Eggs with Cheese

Ingredients

All-purpose flour	2½ tablespoons
Salt	½ teaspoon
Prepared mustard	1 teaspoon
Milk	1½ cups
Butter or margarine	1 tablespoon
Milk cheddar cheese, grated	6 oz
Bread	6 slices
Pepper, cayenne pepper	to taste
Eggs	6

Preparation

Preheat the oven to 350 degrees, 40 minutes before the meal.
Lightly grease six individual baking dishes.
Blend the flour, salt, pepper, cayenne, mustard, and milk, and stir slowly in a saucepan.
Cook until the sauce is thick, and remove from the heat.
Add the butter and cheese, and stir until the sauce is thick and smooth.
Break 1 egg into each dish.
Pour the cheese sauce over the egg (⅓ cup der dish).
Bake 15 to 20 minutes.
Toast the bread and cut into points for each dish.

Portions   6

Exchange Value   1 portion = 2 Meat Exchanges + ½ Milk Exchange + 1 Bread Exchange + 1 Fat Exchange.

Scrambled Eggs and Broccoli

Ingredients

Eggs	4
Skim milk	¼ cup
Salt	¼ teaspoon
Paprika and tabasco	1 pinch
Cooked broccoli, well-drained and chopped	½ cup
Cottage cheese or skim milk cheese	¼ cup
Margarine	2 teaspoons

Beat the eggs and milk in a bowl.
Add the salt and seasonings.
Mix in the broccoli and cheese. Melt the margarine in a frying pan over moderate heat.
Cook the mixture, stirring occasionally, until the eggs are firm but still moist.

Cottage Cheese Omelette

Ingredients

Eggs	**2**
Water	**1 tablespoon**
Cottage cheese	**1 oz**
Salt, pepper, parsley (or chopped chives), marjoram	**to taste**

Preparation

Beat the eggs with the water and seasonings.
Pour into a Teflon frying pan, over moderate heat.
When the underpart of the omelette is set, spoon the cottage cheese onto the middle; fold the omelette and carefully turn it over with the spatula. Slide the omelette onto a warmed plate.

Portion 1

Exchange Value 1 portion = 3 Meat Exchanges.

Variations

1. Substitute processed cheese (1 oz) for cottage cheese. Add 2 Fat Exchanges to the value.
2. Replace the cheese with cooked green peas or onions. The Exchange Value will then be 2 Meat Exchanges + 1 Vegetable Exchange.
3. Substitute canned tomatoes or whole asparagus. Value = 2 Meat Exchanges + ½ Vegetable Exchange.
4. Substitute a bit of green pepper or finely chopped mushrooms. 2 Meat Exchanges.

Macaroni and Cheese

Ingredients	Cooked macaroni, salted and drained	1⅓ cup
	Reconstituted powdered skim milk	½ cup
	Flour	1 tablespoon
	Grated processed cheese	4 oz
	Salt, pepper, green pepper, or mushrooms	to taste

Preparation

Blend the flour in a small amount of water.
Add this to the milk in a double boiler.
Add the cheese and stir as it melts.
When the sauce has thickened, add the spices and condiments.
Pour the sauce over the macaroni in 2 individual baking dishes.
Place in a moderate oven and heat until the top is browned.
Optional: sprinkle each dish with a crumbled Ritz cracker or soda cracker.

Portions

2

Exchange Value

1 portion = 2 Bread Exchanges + 2 Meat Exchanges.

Variation

The exchange value of the recipes can be modified as follows:
½ the amount of macaroni = 1 Bread Exchange.
½ the amount of cheese = 1 Meat Exchange.
Whole milk or butter in the sauce adds ½ Fat Exchange.

Cauliflower with Cheese

Ingredients	Cauliflower	1 large
	Salt	½ teaspoon
	Olive oil	4 teaspoons
	Garlic	1 clove
	Chopped parsley	1 tablespoon
	Grated parmesan cheese	⅓ cup

Preparation

Wash the cauliflower and break into flowerets.
Cook in salted boiling water for 15 to 20 minutes, and drain.
Heat the oil in a thick saucepan.

Sauté the garlic and parsley for about 2 minutes.
Add the cauliflower, and continue to saute for 2 minutes more.
Remove from the heat, and top with grated cheese.

Portions Divide into 4 portions.

Exchange Value 1 portion = 1 Group A Vegetable Exchange + ½ Meat Exchange + 1 Fat Exchange.

Poached Eggs with Mushrooms

Ingredients

Fresh, sliced mushrooms, or well-drained canned mushrooms	**½ lb**
Poached eggs	**4**
Toast	**4 slices**
Butter or margarine	**4 teaspoons**

Preparation Heat the butter or margarine in a frying pan.
Sauté the mushrooms until brown and tender.
Poach the eggs.
Divide the mushrooms between the 4 slices of toast, place the poached eggs on top, and serve immediately.

Portions 4

Exchange Value 1 portion = 1 Bread Exchange + 1 Meat Exchange + 1 Fat Exchange.

vegetables

Vegetables

Vegetables

Be sure to differentiate between Group A Vegetables, Group B vegetables, and the starchy vegetables that are part of the Bread Exchanges.

All of them, whatever their value, lend a distinctive touch to meals, either served separately and unaccompanied, or combined with meat exchanges to create a main course.

Some Clever Ways to Vary the Taste and Look of Vegetables

1. **Seasoning tricks**
   1 or 2 cloves of garlic squeezed onto the vegetables, a few minutes before they're done.
   Parsley or chives (the new freeze-dried kind is handy).
   Lemon, or seasoned vinegar, for a piquant flavor.
   Roasted sesame seeds, or dried celery flakes.
   A pinch of thyme, oregano, or marjoram on tomatoes and green vegetables.
   Tarragon on peas and beets.

2. **Methods of Preparing Before Cooking**
   Broccoli is excellent served whole — or you can eat the flowerets, and save the cooked, tender stalks for another meal.
   A number of vegetables can be easily chopped into cubes, or sliced in thin, Julienne-style sticks. Using a small amount of salted water, considerably reduces the cooking time for potatoes, carrots, turnip, and celery.
   Some vegetables (cabbage, carrots, and turnips) are grated or finely chopped before cooking; other vegetables (e.g. beets) should be cooked first.

3. **Different Ways of Cooking Vegetables**
   Spit-roasted: (shish-ke-bab) Roast on a spit over an outdoor barbecue, or campfire, or on a hibachi. Whatever vegetables

you use should be partially precooked in water, so that they are tender but still firm. Drain and cut into cubes. Large pieces of red or green tomato, eggplant, parsnip, or celery can also be added to the skewer; alternate them with onions of the same size, 4-inch pieces of corn on the cob, and sour pickles. Season with salt and pepper, monosodium glutamate (Accent), and place the skewer about 3 inches above the source of heat, turning slowly. The tomatoes do not need to be precooked.

Broiled: Tomato, celery, onion, summer squash, green pepper, and eggplant are easily broiled in the oven, about 4 inches below the broiler.

Stewed: The same vegetables are ideal for cooking covered in the oven, in a small amount of liquid. This is an excellent way to prepare potatoes, carrots, and all types of squash. Stew the vegetables whole, in cubes, or in thin slices; cooking time will vary according to the size. Invent combinations that please the eye as well as the palate.

Stuffed: Tomatoes, green pepper, and onion are especially suited for this method of cooking. For the stuffing, add one Bread Exchange (⅓ cup cooked rice) to your Meat Exchanges (chicken, shrimp, lobster, etc.) and some butter. Mix together and season to taste.

Steamed: Vegetables cooked by this method, in a covered metal steaming basket, over boiling water, preserve all their natural flavor. Steam them on top of the stove, as described, or in the oven in foil wrap.

Wrapped and Oven-Steamed: Aluminum-wrap portions of vegetables that have been chopped to a consistent size so that they will cook evenly. Season before sealing. The flavor of vegetables cooked in their own juice is exceptional.

Pan-Braising: Place the sliced or cubed vegetables in a pot or thick saucepan, and season well. Add a small amount of good meat stock, with the fat removed. Cover with an air-tight lid and simmer slowly over gentle heat. If the lid does not fit tightly, you can improvise by covering the pot with a sheet of thick aluminum foil. Fold the edges down around the outside of the pot, and place the lid on top. This prevents the steam from escaping.

4. Experiment With Different Vegetables

Steamed leeks—boil shallots or leeks in a small amount of salted water.

Salsify—cooked in boiled water, and salted afterwards. Their oyster flavor is very pleasant.

White turnip—boiled and riced.

Winter squash—steamed and mashed.

Parsnip—cooked in salted boiling water, mashed, and shaped into thin patties; brown in the oven or in a Teflon frying pan.

All these vegetables will be more flavorful if you can add butter, before or after cooking—provided you take into account the extra Fat Exchange. However, all the methods of cooking that we have listed are excellent without butter. Be sure to season them well.

Tomato Aspic

Ingredients		
Unflavored gelatin		1 teaspoon
Cold water		½ cup
Chopped onion		1 teaspoon
Canned tomatoes		½ cup
Chopped celery		1 teaspoon
Cloves		2
Cayenne pepper		several grains
Bay leaf		1
Vinegar		1 tablespoon

Preparation Combine the onion, celery, tomatoes, cloves, cayenne, and bay leaf in a saucepan.
Simmer very gently for ½ an hour, strain, and add 1 tablespoon vinegar.
Dissolve the gelatin in the cold water, and add to the stock.
Stir until thoroughly blended.
Pour into a mould and refrigerate until firm.

Exchange Value Negligible

Variation You can add vegetables (peas, cucumber, celery, etc.) to the aspic when it is partially set. In this case, the Exchange Value = value of the extra vegetables.

Tomato Cocktail

Ingredients		
Lemon		1 slice
Canned tomatoes		2, 28-oz cans
Celery		1 stalk
Carrot		1 medium
Onion salt		½ teaspoon
Bay leaves		2
Saccharine		6 tablets
Salt and pepper		to taste

Preparation   Combine the tomatoes, celery, carrot, onion salt, saccharine, and bay leaves in a pot.
Simmer gently for one hour, adding water if necessary.
Continue to simmer another hour; add salt and pepper to taste.
Strain the liquid, crushing the vegetables to extract all the juice.
Serve cold, with a slice of lemon.

Portions   6, 4-oz servings

Exchange Value   1 portion = 1 Group A Vegetable Exchange.

Note   This cocktail is even better when prepared several days ahead.

Stewed Celery

Ingredients		
Chicken stock	**½ cup**	
Celery, coarsely chopped	**3 cups**	
Onion, thinly sliced	**¼ cup**	
Apple, unpeeled, cut into thin slices	**½ medium**	

Preparation   Place all the ingredients except the apple in a saucepan.
Bring to a boil.
Cover and simmer 5 minutes, or until the celery is tender.
Add the sliced apple, and cook 5 minutes.

Portions   4, ½ cup servings.

Exchange Value   1 portion = 1 Group A Vegetable Exchange, or ½ Fruit Exchange.

Stuffed Celery

Ingredients	Celery	8 large 12″ stalks
	Sesame seeds	¼ cup
	Cottage cheese	8 oz
	Onion salt	¼ teaspoon

Preparation

Preheat the oven to 350 degrees.

Spread the sesame seeds on a baking sheet, and roast for 5 to 10 minutes.

Blend the cottage cheese with the onion salt with an electric mixer. Fill the celery stalks evenly with the mixture, and sprinkle with the roasted seeds.

Cut each stalk into 4 pieces, and keep crisp and firm in the refrigerator.

Portions   8

Exchange Value

4 pieces, or 1 stalk = 1 Group A Vegetable Exchange
+ 1 Meat Exchange.

Carrots with Orange

Ingredients	Carrots, peeled and cut in thin diagonal slices 6 medium
	Butter or margarine 2 tablespoons
	Orange sections 4 medium sections
	Sugar substitute equivalent to
	2 tablespoons

Preparation

Cook the carrots in salted boiling water.
Drain, add the butter, orange and sugar substitute, and reheat.

Portions   4

Exchange Value

1 Group B Vegetable Exchange + 1 Fruit Exchange + 1 Fat Exchange.

Green Beans with Mint

Ingredients	Canned or frozen green beans	16 oz (packaged or canned)
	Dried mint (in gauze bag)	¼ cup
	Butter	2 tablespoons
	Salt and pepper	to taste

Preparation Bring the beans and mint to the point of boiling, add the butter, and season with salt and pepper.

Portions 6

Exchange Value 1 portion = 1 Group A Vegetable Exchange + 1 Fat Exchange.

Yellow Beans, Italian Style

Ingredients	Yellow beans	1 lb
	Tomato juice	1 cup
	Garlic	1 clove
	Salt and pepper	to taste

Preparation Cook the beans in salted water and drain them well.
Add the tomato juice and pressed garlic, season with salt and pepper.
Simmer 10 minutes.

Portions 4

Exchange Value 1 portion = 1 Group A Vegetable Exchange

Salad Plate

A plain salad can be easily transformed into a complete meal.

On a generous bed of fresh lettuce, arrange the six varieties of vegetables that form the basic ingredients of a salad.

1. **Celery — cut into plain sticks, or decorative curled ones.**
2. **Medium tomato — sliced or in quarters.**
3. **Cucumber — 4 medium slices**
4. **Shallots — 2 or 3 small**
5. **Radish — 4**
6. **Peas — 2 tablespoons**

At this stage, the Exchange Value of an individual salad = 1 Group A (5% or less) Vegetable Exchange + 1 Group B (10% or less) Vegetable Exchange.

To complete the salad, add your choice of:

— Sliced hard-boiled eggs	1 = 1 Meat Exchange
— 1 hard-boiled egg, plus 1, 1-oz slice of meat	= 2 Meat Exchanges
— 1 hard-boiled egg, plus 1, 1-oz slice of meat plus 1, 1-oz slice of processed cheese	= 3 Meat Exchanges
— ¼ cup canned salmon, tuna, or lobster, well-drained	= 1 Meat Exchange
— 5 shrimps	= 1 Meat Exchange
— additional portion of Potato Salad (see recipe in chapter on Starchy Foods)	= 1 Bread Exchange + 1 Fat Exchange
— Oil and Vinegar, or Mayonnaise, from the chapter on sauces	= negligible value, or whatever value is indicated.
— Five small olives	= 1 Fat Exchange

Note that the salad can include almost all the food exchanges, according to your taste. With all its variations, the Salad Plate offers plenty of possibilities for a mealtime change of pace.

Waldorf Salad

Ingredients		
	Diced celery	¼ cup
	Diced apple, sprinkled with lemon juice	1 small
	Special Salad Dressing (see chapter on sauces)	small amount
	Paprika	1 pinch

Preparation
Combine the celery and the apple.
Arrange on a lettuce leaf, and top with a bit of salad dressing; dust with paprika.

Portion
1

Exchange Value
1 portion = 1 Fruit Exchange or 1 Group B Vegetable Exchange.

Green Salad

Ingredients
Your choice of these fresh vegetable combinations:
— **lettuce, cucumber, celery, green pepper**
— **endive with tomato or cucumber**
— **chicory, tomato, radish**
— **cabbage, celery, green pepper**
— **lettuce, watercress, with or without cucumber**
— **lettuce, spinach greens, with or without radish**

Preparation
Wash, dry, and trim the vegetables.
Tear the lettuce, or chop the cabbage, and chop the other vegetables.
Combine in a salad bowl.
Season with salt, pepper, etc., and vinegar or lemon juice.

Exchange Value
1 large bowl = negligible value, or 1 Group A Vegetable Exchange.

Variation
Accompany either with Zero Mayonnaise, or the Special Salad Dressing (see chapter on sauces), adding on the exchange values indicated.

Cabbage Salad

Ingredients		
	Cider vinegar	3 tablespoons
	Salad oil	4 teaspoons
	Chopped parsley	1 tablespoon
	Salt and pepper	¼ teaspoon
	Dried mustard	½ teaspoon
	Chopped cabbage	¼
	Diced carrots, drained	1 cup (canned)
	French-style green beans	1 cup (canned)
	Diced green pepper	1
	Chopped onion	¼ cup

Preparation Mix together the vinegar, oil, and seasonings in the salad bowl. Add the vegetables, and mix carefully.

Portions Divide into 4 portions.

Exchange Value 1 portion = 1 Group B Vegetable Exchange + 1 Fat Exchange.

Newfangled Salad

Ingredients		
	Diced green pepper	1
	Tomato in quarters	1 medium
	Apple, washed and sliced thinly	1 small
	Celery, chopped in small pieces	2 stalks
	Chopped parsley	2 tablespoons
	Ordinary mayonnaise	4 teaspoons
	Lemon juice	½ tablespoon

Preparation Combine all the ingredients.

Portions Divide into 4 portions

Exchange Value 1 portion = 1 Group B Vegetable Exchange + 1 Fat Exchange.

Chef Salad

Ingredients		
Lettuce, torn into fairly small pieces		**1 head**
Tomatoes, cut in sections		**2**
Garlic		**1 clove**
Salt and pepper		**to taste**

Preparation

Rub the salad bowl with the clove of garlic.
Tear the lettuce, leaf by leaf; add the tomatoes and seasonings.
Toss gently.

Portions

4

Exchange Value

1 portion = 1 Group A Vegetable Exchange.

desserts

pie-fillings, puddings and punch
fruit preserves without sugar
fruit plates

Desserts

**Pie-fillings, Puddings and Punch
Fruit Preserves Without Sugar**

Desserts

When you're restricted to a calculated diet, the last course of a meal usually consists of fruit (10% value), eaten plain. But fruit can also be combined with all the exchanges—bread, milk, fat, or meat, depending on the dish. If you've been resigned to leaving the dinner table after the main course is over, read on; with fruit, or mousse, or a meringue, you can end the meal with a flourish.

As proof positive that a diabetic diet doesn't have to be bland and colorless, we offer you a number of surprising desserts—not all of them based on fruit, either—to brighten your mealtimes.

Ambrosia Fruit Cup

Ingredients	Whole orange, sliced	small
	Half a banana, sliced	medium
	Grated coconut	4 tablespoons

Preparation Combine the sliced fruit.
Add 2 tablespoons water sweetened with sugar substitute (optional).
Divide equally between 2 dessert cups, and sprinkle each with 2 tablespoons coconut.

Portions 2

Exchange Value 1 portion = 1 Fruit Exchange + 1 Fat Exchange.

Apple Mousse

Ingredients	Apple sauce, unsweetened	1½ cups
	Evaporated milk, very cold	¾ cup
	Lemon juice	1½ teaspoons
	Salt	1 pinch
	Nutmeg	1 pinch

Preparation Beat the evaporated milk until it becomes firm.
Fold in the rest of the ingredients.
Pour into 3 bowls and leave until firm.

Portions 3

Exchange Value 1 portion = 1 Fruit Exchange + ½ Milk Exchange.

Apricot Mousse

Ingredients	Eggwhites	2
	Salt	⅛ teaspoon
	Canned apricots—	
	sugar-free diet variety, or	
	the regular canned variety, drained	16 oz
	Sugar substitute	optional

Preparation Beat the egg whites until stiff, sprinkling in the salt.
Blend the apricots to a purée consistency, and fold into the whites.

Portions Divide into 5 portions

Exchange Value 1 portion = 1 Fruit Exchange.

Banana Mousse

Ingredients	Unflavored gelatin	1 tablespoon
	Cold water	¼ cup
	Boiling water	⅓ cup
	Lemon juice	2 tablespoons
	Sugar substitute	optional
	Bananas, mashed	⅔ cup
	Egg whites, beaten	2

Preparation Soak the gelatin in the cold water, then add to the boiling water,
along with the juice.
Stir until thoroughly dissolved.
Refrigerate until partially set, then add the mashed bananas
and beat until spongy.
Fold in the stiff egg whites, and beat just enough to blend
the ingredients.

Portions Divide equally in 6 half-cup portions

Exchange Value 1 portion = 1 Fruit Exchange.

Bavarian Ice Cream

Ingredients	Sugar-free gelatin (D'Zerta)—	
	orange-lime, strawberry, or raspberry	**2 tablespoons**
	Boiling water	**2 cups**
	Vanilla ice cream	**1 pint**

Preparation Dissolve the gelatin in the boiling water.
Chill until partially set.
Let the pint of ice cream soften at room temperature for about 5 minutes; cut up and add to the gelatin.
Beat with an electric mixer until the ice cream is melted.

Portions Pour into 6 cups.

Exchange Value 1 portion = 1 Fruit Exchange + 1 Fat Exchange.

Blancmange

Ingredients	**Milk**	**1 cup**
	Cornstarch	**1 level tablespoon**
	Salt	**1 pinch**
	Sugar substitute	**¼ teaspoon**
	Vanilla	**1 teaspoon**

Preparation Heat ¾ cup of milk to the boiling point, in a double boiler.
Blend the cornstarch in ¼ cup of cold milk, and add this mixture to the hot milk.
Cook for 20 minutes, or until the starchy taste is gone.
Add the salt, sugar substitute, and vanilla.

Portions Divide equally in 2 dessert cups.

Exchange Value 1 portion (half the recipe) = ½ Milk Exchange.

Chocolate Mousse

Ingredients		
	Gelatin	1 tablespoon
	Cold water	¼ cup
	Warm milk	1½ cups
	Bitter chocolate	1½ oz
	Boiling water	¼ cup
	Vanilla	1 teaspoon
	Egg whites	2
	Sugar substitute	to taste

Preparation
Soak the gelatin in the cold water, then dissolve in the warm milk.
Melt the chocolate over hot water.
Add the suger substitute, gradually pour in the boiling water,
and flavor with the vanilla.
Mix this into the milk and gelatin mixture.
Let cool, stirring occasionally.
When the mixture is partially set, whip till frothy.
Beat the egg whites until they form stiff peaks, and gently fold
into the chocolate mixture.
Pour into a mold and chill.

Portions   6

**Exchange
Value**   1 portion = ½ Fruit Exchange + 1 Fat Exchange.

Christmas Meringues

Ingredients		
	Egg whites	4
	Salt	½ teaspoon
	Cream of tartar	1 teaspoon
	Vanilla, or other flavoring extract	½ teaspoon
	Liquid sugar substitute equivalent to	1 cup of sugar

Preparation
Preheat the oven to 250 degrees.
Let the egg whites reach room temperature.
Make sure that your mixing bowl and electric beaters have no trace
of grease or water on them; wipe with a dry towel.

Beat the egg whites, while adding the salt and cream of tartar, until stiff.

As soon as the whites will form stiff, glossy peaks, stop beating, and add the sugar substitute.

Cover a baking sheet with brown paper on which you've drawn Christmas motifs—bells, trees, Santas, etc.

Spoon the meringue onto the paper, keeping within the outlines.

Cook the meringues **very slowly** for 1¼ hours.

When they are done, they will be golden, dry and crunchy on the outside, and slightly moist in the centre.

Serve as an accompaniment for a fruit dessert, or as a special treat any time.

Exchange Value   None

Crème Bartlett

Ingredients		
Egg yolks		4
Skim milk		1½ cups
Orange peel, grated		2 teaspoons
Sugar substitute		to taste
Salt		1 pinch
Almond extract		¼ teaspoon
Canned, unsweetened pears, drained		4 halves
Unsweetened fruit salad, drained		1 cup

Preparation

Lightly beat the 4 egg yolks in a medium-sized saucepan.

Gradually add the skim milk.

Cook over low heat, stirring continually, until the mixture will coat a spoon.

Remove from the heat, and add the orange peel, sugar substitute, salt, and almond extract.

Refrigerate until cool but not set.

Place one pear half in a sherbet dish, and pour ¼ of the custard over it.

Refrigerate the four desserts, and just before serving, top each with ¼ cup chilled fruit salad.

Portions	4
Exchange Value	1 portion = 1 Fruit Exchange + 1 Meat Exchange.

Diet Gelatin, Any Flavor

Ingredients	Unflavored gelatin	1 teaspoon
	Cold water	2 tablespoons
	Boiling water	½ cup
	Lemon juice	1 tablespoon

Preparation Soak the gelatin in the cold water for 10 minutes.
Add the lemon juice to the boiling water, and pour into the gelatin; stir until completely dissolved.
Pour into an individual-portion mold, and chill until set.

Portions 1

Exchange Value Negligible

Variations: **Coffee gelatin:** Leave out the lemon, and replace the half-cup water with an equal amount of coffee.
Chocolate Gelatin: Omit the lemon, and blend 1 teaspoon cocoa in a bit of cold water; add last.
Extracts: Add a drop of almond extract, or extract of rum, mint, coconut, strawberry, pineapple, etc.
Fruit Gelatin: Replace the half-cup boiling water with an equal amount of unsweetened fruit juice. In this case, exchange value = 1 Fruit Exchange.

Whipped Cream Substitute

Ingredients		
	Cold water	¼ cup
	Powdered skim milk	3 tablespoons
	Sugar substitute equivalent to	½ cup sugar
	Lemon juice	1 tablespoon

Preparation
Chill all the ingredients.
Place the bowl and beaters in the refrigerator as well.
Combine all the ingredients in the chilled bowl, and beat with an electric mixer, at top speed, until peaks form.
Make this just before serving, and use right away.

Portions
1 cup

Exchange Value
Negligible

Fruit Cocktail

Ingredients		
	1 peach half, canned, unsweetened	
	1 pear half, canned, unsweetened	
	Half an apple	medium
	Half an orange	medium
	Half a banana	small
	Grapes (Malaga), pitted and halved	6
	Sugar substitute equivalent to	3 tablespoons sugar
	Water	1 cup
	Lemon juice	1 tablespoon

Preparation
Make a syrup by boiling the water with the sugar substitute.
Flavor with the lemon juice.
Dice and combine the fruit, and pour the syrup over it.
Cover the bowl with Saran Wrap, and chill in the refrigerator.

Portions
Divide equally between 3 bowls or dessert cups.

Exchange Value
1 portion = 1 Fruit Exchange.

Fruit Gelatin

Ingredients	Orange juice	1 cup
	Boiling water	1 cup
	Lemon juice	1 tablespoon
	Unflavored gelatin	1 tablespoon

Preparation Combine the orange juice and lemon juice.
Add the gelatin and put aside for a few minutes.
Add the boiling water, stir, and let chill.

Portions Divide into 4 equal parts of a half-cup each.

Exchange Value 1 portion = ½ Fruit Exchange.

Junket

Ingredients	Junket	1 tablet
	Cold water	1 tablespoon
	Fresh milk, warm	2 cups
	Sugar substitute equivalent to	3 tablespoons sugar
	Extract of vanilla, or orange, lemon, strawberry, etc.	1 teaspoon

Preparation Dissolve the tablet of junket in the cold water.
Briefly warm the milk, and add the junket.
Add the sugar substitute and the extract.
Stir thoroughly, and pour at once into 4 bowls.
Do not stir again. Leave undisturbed until set.

Portions 4

Exchange Value 1 portion or 1 bowl = ½ Milk Exchange.

Lemon Mousse

Ingredients		
Cold water		¼ cup
Unflavored gelatin		2 tablespoons
Eggs (room temperature)		5
Salt		⅛ teaspoon
Sugar substitute equivalent to		¾ cup sugar
Lemon juice		¼ cup
Lemon peel, grated		2 teaspoons

Preparation Soak the gelatin in the cold water.
Stir over low heat until the gelatin is dissolved.
Chill.
Use the top speed of your electric mixer, and a large bowl,
to beat the egg whites.
Beat, while adding the salt, until the whites form peaks.
In a small bowl, combine the egg yolks and sugar substitute,
and beat at high speed for about 5 minutes, or until the yolks
are thick and lemon colored.
At a lower speed, beat in the lemon juice, grated peel, and gelatin.
Gently fold this mixture into the egg whites.

Portions Spoon into 6 dessert dishes.

Exchange Value 1 portion = 1 Meat Exchange.

Mocha Mousse

Ingredients		
Gelatin		1 tablespoon
Cold water		½ cup
Sugar substitute equivalent to ⅓ cup sugar, plus enough water to make		¼ cup
Salt		⅛ teaspoon
Boiling water		1 cup
Cocoa		2 teaspoons
Instant coffee		½ teaspoon

Preparation   Soak the gelatin in the cold water, in a medium-sized bowl.
Add the other ingredients, and stir until the gelatin is thoroughly dissolved.
Use an egg beater or electric mixer to beat until the mixture is light and frothy.

Portions   6

Exchange Value   1 daily portion = none.

No-Pastry Apple Pie

Ingredients

Cooking apples, peeled and sliced thin	4 apples
Unflavored gelatin	1 envelope
Lemon juice	3 tablespoons
Powdered skim milk	⅔ cup
Water	1½ cups
Cinnamon	½ teaspoon
Sugar substitute equivalent to	4 teaspoons sugar

Preparation   Preheat the oven to 350 degrees.
Place the apple slices in a 9'' pie plate.
In a small bowl, combine the lemon juice, gelatin, sugar substitute, and the water. Stir well.
Pour this mixture over the apple slices.
Spread the powdered milk mixed with the cinnamon on top.
Cook 1 hour, or until the apples are tender.
Refrigerate overnight.

Portions   Divide into 8 portions.

Exchange Value   1 portion = 1 Fruit Exchange.

Orange-Apple Cocktail

Ingredients   Medium orange
Small apple

Preparation   Peel and cut up the orange.
Wash and dice the apple; sprinkle with lemon juice.

Portions   Divide equally in 2 bowls.

**Exchange
Value**   1 portion, or ½ cup = 1 Fruit Exchange.

Orange Jelly

Ingredients   Diet Gelatin, orange-flavored (see recipe in this chapter).
Half an orange, in sections.

Preparation   Place the orange sections in a dessert dish.
Prepare the diet gelatin.
When the gelatin is half set, pour into the dish and chill
until completely firm.

Portions   1 dessert dish

**Exchange
Value**   1 dish = ½ Fruit Exchange.

Variation   When serving, garnish with 2 tablespoons of special whipped
cream, prepared as follows.
Blend well with a mixer: ½ cup cold water, 1 tablespoon lemon
juice, 5 tablespoons skim milk powder. Yields 12 portions.

Orange Parfait

Ingredients   Unflavored gelatin   1 tablespoon
Unsweetened orange juice   2 cups
Vanilla ice cream, softened   1 cup
Liquid sugar substitute
Orange extract   ¼ teaspoon
Red food coloring   3 drops
Yellow food coloring   2 drops

Preparation	Pour the orange juice into a saucepan, add the gelatin, and stir over low heat until thoroughly dissolved.
	Remove from the heat, and mix in the other ingredients.
	Refrigerate until partially set.
	Whip the mixture, and pour into 6 individual molds.
	Return to the refrigerator until completely firm.

Portions 6

**Exchange
Value** 1 portion = 1 Bread Exchange + 1 Fat Exchange.

Orange Pudding

Ingredients	Whole milk	2½ cups
	Orange peel, grated (of 1 orange)	
	Cornstarch	3 tablespoons
	Liquid sugar substitute	
	Salt	1 pinch
	Eggs, separated	3
	Vanilla	1 teaspoon

Preparation Heat 2 cups of milk, with the orange peel added, to the boiling point.
Combine the cornstarch, salt, and sugar substitute in ½ cup cold milk.
Pour this into the warm milk, and cook in the double boiler, stirring, until it begins to thicken.
Cover and continue cooking about 30 minutes.
Add the beaten egg yolks, stir until smooth, and cook 2 or 3 minutes.
Flavor with vanilla.
Pour into a mold, and cover with the egg whites which have been beaten until stiff.
Place in a 300-degree oven just long enough to brown the meringue.

Portions Divide into 6 equal portions.

**Exchange
Value** 1 portion = 1 Fruit Exchange + 1 Meat Exchange.

Peach Amandine

Ingredients		
	Canned peaches, unsweetened	8 halves
	Skim milk, fresh or reconstituted	½ cup
	Almond extract	½ teaspoon
	Creamed cottage cheese	4 oz

Preparation
Blend the milk and cottage cheese into a sauce.
Flavor with the almond extract.
Divide the peach halves between 4 dessert bowls.
Pour the sauce over them, and top each with half a maraschino cherry and a mint leaf.
Chill and serve.

Portions 4

Exchange Value 1 portion = 1 Fruit Exchange + 1 Meat Exchange

Peach Cobbler

Ingredients		
	Cornstarch	½ tablespoon
	Cold water	½ cup
	Sugar substitute equivalent to	½ cup sugar
	Peaches, peeled and sliced; or apples, pears, or plums	4 cups
	Premixed biscuit dough (Bisquick)	1 cup
	Salt	½ teaspoon
	Coffee cream	½ cup
	Vanilla	½ teaspoon
	Grated lemon peel	1 teaspoon
	Sugar substitute equivalent to	2 tablespoons sugar

Preparation
Preheat the oven to 425 degrees.
Blend the cornstarch in the half-cup water.
Add the sugar substitute and the fruit.
Pour into an ovenproof serving dish or casserole.
Combine the other ingredients and mix into a dough.
Spread the dough on top of the fruit, and bake, uncovered, for about 40 minutes.

Portions	Divide into 8 equal portions.
Exchange Value	1 portion = 1 Bread Exchange + 1 Fat Exchange + 1 Fruit Exchange.

Peach Flan

Ingredients	Unflavored gelatin	1 tablespoon (1 envelope)
	Cold water	2 tablespoons
	Warm water	¼ cup
	Vanilla	½ teaspoon
	Sugar substitute equivalent to	¼ cup sugar
	Unsweetened peaches	4 halves
	Whole milk	1 cup
	Powdered skim milk	¼ cup

Preparation	Soak the gelatin in the water, then dissolve thoroughly in the warm water. Add the other ingredients and stir a few seconds.
Portions	Pour into 4 cups.
Exchange Value	1 portion = 1 Fruit Exchange + ½ Meat Exchange.

Peach Melba

Ingredients	Canned peaches, unsweetened	4 halves
	Vanilla ice cream	4 scoops (⅓ cup)
	Diet raspberry syrup (see below)	1 cup

Preparation	Place one peach half, with a scoop of ice cream in the hollow of it, in each bowl. Top with ¼ cup raspberry syrup per portion, and serve immediately.
Portions	4
Exchange Value	1 portion = 1 Fruit Exchange + 1 Group A Vegetable Exchange + 1 Fat Exchange.

Raspberry Syrup: Thaw and drain 1 package frozen, unsweetened raspberries. Add enough water to the melted juice to make 1 cup liquid. Bring the juice to a boil, and thicken with 1 tablespoon cornstarch. Sweeten to taste with a sugar substitute, and let cool.

Peach-Orange Sherbet

Ingredients		
Unsweetened peaches, blended or mashed to a smooth consistency		**1¾ cups**
Sugar substitute equivalent to ½ cup sugar, plus enough water to make		**¼ cup**
Grapefruit juice, unsweetened		**¼ cup**
Orange juice, unsweetened		**½ cup**
Lemon juice		**1 tablespoon**
Egg whites, beaten till stiff		**2**

Preparation

Combine the peach purée, fruit juices, and the water with sugar substitute.

Pour into a dish, and place in the freezer until the mixture is frozen for an inch around the edge, but not in the centre.

At the same time, chill another bowl of the same size.

Pour the fruit mixture into the chilled bowl and beat with an electric mixer.

Fold in the stiff egg whites.

Return to the freezer and chill until firm.

If the sherbet is too hard, let it thaw slowly, beat it again, and refreeze at a warmer temperature.

Portions

Divide in 6 portions of a half cup each.

Exchange Value

1 portion = 1 Fruit Exchange.

Pineapple Tapioca

Ingredients	Minute tapioca	1 tablespoon
	Pineapple juice, unsweetened	3 oz
	Water	1 tablespoon
Preparation	Combine the 3 ingredients and bring to a boil.	
	Cook for 2 minutes, remove from the heat, and let cool.	
	Pour into a bowl, and decorate with two small chunks of pineapple.	
Portions	1	
Exchange Value	1 portion = 1 Fruit Exchange + 1 Group B Vegetable Exchange.	
	or = 2 Fruit Exchanges.	

Rice Pudding

Ingredients	Egg	1
	Milk	¾ cup
	Salt	1 pinch
	Cooked rice	3 tablespoons
	Vanilla	⅛ teaspoon
	Liquid sugar substitute	
Preparation	Beat the egg, and add the milk, salt, vanilla, and rice.	
	Pour into 2 molds and place in a pan of warm water.	
	Bake in a moderate oven (300 degrees) for an hour.	
Portions	2	
Exchange Value	1 portion = 1 Fruit Exchange + 1 Meat Exchange.	

Snow Pudding

Ingredients		
Gelatin		1½ teaspoons
Cold water		1 tablespoon
Boiling water		⅔ cup
Egg white		1
Lemon juice		3 tablespoons
Sugar substitute		

Preparation
Soak the gelatin in the cold water.
Add the boiling water, and stir until the gelatin is dissolved.
Add the lemon juice and sugar substitute.
Let the pudding partially set, then fold in the stiffly beaten egg white.

Portions
Spoon into 3 molds.

Exchange Value
1 portion = none.

Spanish Cream

Ingredients		
Unflavored gelatin		1½ tablespoons
Cold water		1½ tablespoons
1 egg, separated		
Warm milk		1 cup
Liquid sugar substitute		
Vanilla		¼ teaspoon (optional)

Preparation
Soak the gelatin in the cold water.
Lightly beat the egg yolk, and add to the warm milk.
Cook in a double boiler until the egg thickens.
Add the gelatin, and stir thoroughly till dissolved.
Remove from the heat, add the sugar substitute, and flavor with vanilla.
Beat the egg white until stiff, and fold into the custard.
Serve chilled.

Portions
Divide into 3 portions.

Exchange Value	1 portion = ½ Meat Exchange.
Variation	The quantity of fruit allowed for the meal, can be added as garnish.

Special Icing

Ingredients	Diet gelatin (D'Zerta), strawberry or raspberry	1 envelope
Preparation	To obtain a creamy, pale pink icing for any cake, let the gelatin partially set, and then beat until fluffy.	
Exchange Value	None	

Special Yogurt

Ingredients	Plain yogurt	6 oz
	Canned mandarin oranges, unsweetened, well drained, and cut into pieces	½ cup
	Almond extract	½ teaspoon
Preparation	Use an electric mixer to combine the ingredients, and chill.	
Portions	Divide between 2 bowls.	
Exchange Value	1 portion = ½ Meat Exchange + 1 Fruit Exchange.	

Stewed Rhubarb and Strawberries

Ingredients	Frozen, unsweetened strawberries	1 cup
	Frozen, unsweetened rhubarb	1 cup
	Sugar substitute	
Preparation	Combine and cook for 5 minutes.	
Portions	4 half-cup servings	
Exchange Value	1 portion = ½ Fruit Exchange.	

Strawberry-Banana Cocktail

Ingredients	Banana	½
	Unsweetened strawberries	¾ cup

Preparation Mix the strawberries and sliced bananas in a bowl.

Portions Divide equally in 2 dishes.

Exchange Value 1 portion, or ½ cup = 1 Fruit Exchange.

Strawberry Cream

Ingredients	Skim milk, fresh or reconstituted	1 cup
	Frozen, unsweetened strawberries	1½ cups
	1 egg	
	Vanilla	1 teaspoon
	Sugar substitute	to taste

Preparation Mix all ingredients in a blender at high speed, about 5 seconds.

Portions Divide equally in 2 bowls.

Exchange Value 1 portion = 1 Fruit Exchange + ½ Meat Exchange.

Strawberry Snow

Ingredients	Egg whites	2
	Cream of tartar	¼ teaspoon
	Salt	1 pinch
	Fresh or frozen strawberries, unsweetened, sliced	1½ cups
	Sugar substitute	optional

Preparation Whip the egg whites until stiff, while adding the salt and cream of tartar.
Carefully fold in the strawberries.
Add sugar substitute, if desired.

Portions	Divide in 2 dessert cups.
Exchange Value	1 portion = 1 Fruit Exchange.

Apple Jelly

Ingredients	Lemon juice	1 tablespoon
	Cornstarch	1 teaspoon
	Apple juice, unsweetened	1 cup
	Sugar substitute equivalent to	1 cup sugar
	Unflavored gelatin	1 teaspoon
	Salt	1 pinch

Preparation

Combine the lemon juice, gelatin, cornstarch, and salt in a saucepan; blend until smooth.
Add the apple juice.
Heat, stirring constantly, until it reaches a full boil.
Simmer 2 minutes.
Remove from the heat, and add the sugar substitute.
Let cool.

Exchange Value

2 tablespoons = ½ Fruit Exchange.

Lemon Pie Filling (1)

Ingredients	Lemon diet gelatin (D'Zerta)	2 envelopes
	Egg whites, beaten till stiff	2
	Sugar substitute	to taste
	Cream of tartar	½ teaspoon
	Precooked piecrust	

Preparation

Prepare the D'Zerta as indicated on the package.
Let it set partially.
Whip this mixture and pour into the precooked pie crust.
Beat the egg whites until stiff, while adding the sugar substitute and cream of tartar, and top the filling with this.

Exchange Value

None (for the filling)

Lemon Pie Filling (2)

Ingredients		
	Unflavored gelatin	4½ teaspoons
	Cold water	3 tablespoons
	Boiling water	2 cups
	Egg whites	3
	Lemon juice	9 tablespoons
	Sugar substitute	
	Precooked piecrust	

Preparation

Soak the gelatin in the cold water.
Add the boiling water, and stir until completely dissolved.
Add the lemon juice and sugar substitute.
Leave until partially set.
Beat the egg whites until they will form peaks.
Fold these into the lemon mixture, and pour the filling into the piecrust.

Exchange Value

None (for the filling)

Pineapple Punch

Ingredients		
	Cold tea	¾ cup
	Pineapple juice, unsweetened	3 tablespoons
	Lemon juice	1 tablespoon
	Liquid sugar substitute	

Preparation

Combine everything ahead of time, and serve over ice cubes.

Portions

2, 4-oz servings

Exchange Value

1 portion = negligible value.

Sparkling Punch

Ingredients	**Fresh or frozen orange juice, unsweetened**	**2 cups**
	Peppermint extract	**¼ teaspoon**
	Red food coloring	

Preparation   Mix well and chill.

Exchange Value   1, 4-oz serving = 1 Fruit Exchange.

Sugar-free Fruit Preserves

Necessary Equipment
— Glass Mason jars, in perfect condition (no chips or cracks); these usually have a one-pint capacity.
— Metal lids: with 2 parts, a metal ring that screws tightly onto the jar, and a metal disc with a rubber ring to ensure a good seal.
— A small saucepan.
— A large preserving kettle with an airtight lid, and a metal basket or rack inside, to keep the jars from hitting the bottom and cracking.
— A medium saucepan for fruit that has to be precooked.
— a ladle, tongs, and slotted spoon.
— A deep roasting pan to put the jars in after sterilizing.

Preparing the Jars
Wash the jars in soapy boiling water, and rinse them thoroughly to avoid any trace of soap residue.
Place the jars in the preserving kettle, cover them with boiling water, and keep hot until you need them.
Put the lids, minus the rubber rings, in a small saucepan of water and boil them. Keep them in boiling water too until needed.
The rubber linings should be carefully washed but not boiled, and left in warm rinse water.

Preparing the Fruit
Choose fruit in perfect condition — fresh, firm, and not over-ripe.
Prepare the fruit according to the particular method described in the Preparation Table that follows.
During preparation, place the fruit in water that has a small amount of lemon juice or salt in it, to prevent discoloration that exposure to air causes.
Drain the fruit, place it in a saucepan with some water, and cook slowly for the length of time indicated in the Table.
After cooking, remove the fruit from the water and immediately put them into the hot sterilized jars.
Fill the jars until the fruit is precisely ½ an inch from the top.

Pour the cooking liquid over the fruit, to the same level (½ inch from the top).

Berries or small fruit — blueberries, raspberries, etc. — do not require precooking.

Wipe the edge of the jars with a clean towel.

While the metal circle is still very hot, place it on top of the jar and firmly screw on the hot metal ring.

Note: It is important that the jar, fruit, and lid all be kept hot during the procedure.

Sterilization

When the jars are full and tightly sealed, place them on the wire rack, or in the basket of the large preserving kettle, filled with boiling water.

Make sure an inch of water covers the jar, and put the lid on the kettle.

Count the sterilizing time according to the type of fruit (see Table), and start from the point where the water around the jars reaches a fast boil.

Add boiling water as needed, to maintain the same level of water; the boiling point should remain constant.

When the boiling period is over, take the jars out of the kettle and place them standing, right side up, on a wooden board, preferably covered with a layer of cloth (woollen blanket, eiderdown, etc.).

Leave the jars to cool somewhere where they won't be disturbed by drafts; if they are chilled suddenly, the jars may crack. Store the fruit in a cool, dark spot. Warmth and light can discolor the fruit, and even adversely affect preservation.

All canned fruit has the same value as a similar portion of fresh fruit. For example: 2 peach halves, preserved, are equal to a fresh peach, or one fruit exchange.

We strongly suggest that you do not add any sugar substitute when preserving fruit. If you like a sweeter flavor than what is naturally produced by the fruit, liquid sugar substitute can be added just before serving.

PREPARATION TABLE FOR PRESERVING FRUIT

Fruit	Preparation	Cooking Time	Sterilizing Time
Apples	Wash, peel, cut into pieces	4 min.	25 min.
Berries	Remove stems, wash, sort	none	20 min.
Cherries	remove stems, wash, drain	4 min.	20 min.
Grapes	Wash, drain, sort	3 min.	20 min.
Peaches	Wash, peel, slice, and remove pits	4 min.	20 min.
Pears	Wash, peel, quarter	5 min.	20 min.
Pineapples	Peel, cut into slices or cubes	8 min.	30 min.
Plums	Wash, do not peel; prick the skin in 4 or 5 places	5 min.	20 min.

Fruit Plate (1)

Wash and drain the fruit well; place on a plate lined with lots of fresh, crisp lettuce leaves.

Pineapple, unsweetened	**1 slice**
Prunes, "	**2**
Pear, "	**½**
Peach, "	**½**
Fresh grapes	**6 medium**
Diet gelatin, fruit-flavored	**optional**

Exchange Value: 1 Group A Vegetable Exchange + 1 Group B
Vegetable Exchange + 1 Fruit Exchange.

Supplement with:
¼ cup cottage cheese = 1 Meat Exchange
1 oz cheddar cheese = 1 Meat Exchange
1 oz skim milk cheese = 1 Meat Exchange

Fruit Plate (2)

Place on a fresh bed of lettuce:
1 small orange, quartered or sliced
1 small red apple, unpeeled, and sliced thin
¼ small grapefruit, in sections or sliced

Exchange Value: 1 Group A Vegetable Exchange + 1 Group B
Vegetable Exchange + 1 Fruit Exchange.

Fruit Plate (3)

Prepare as for Plates 1 and 2, and add a small banana.
Increase Exchange Value by 1 Bread Exchange.

Fruit Plate (4)

Place the following on a generous bed of fresh lettuce:
1 small fresh pear, quartered
1 medium-sized fresh peach, quartered
½ cup fresh strawberries
Garnish, if you wish, with Diet Gelatin, fruit-flavored

Exchange Value: 1 Group A Vegetable Exchange + 1 Group B
Vegetable Exchange + 1 Fruit Exchange.

Accompany with a fruit sauce (see chapter on sauces)
or a tablespoon of whipped cream (= 1 Fat Exchange)
or 2 tablespoons of light cream (= 2 Fat Exchanges)

starchy foods

Starchy Foods

Starchy Foods

These include Bread Exchanges eaten by themselves, or used as ingredients in soups, vegetable dishes, main courses, or desserts.

Starches have the advantage of being extremely versatile — as long as you keep their exchange values in mind when you prepare your daily meal plan.

The Potato

Economic, nutritious, good-tasting, and easy to digest . . . there are plenty of obvious virtues to justify the popularity of the potato. The bonus is the number of different ways you can prepare this food.

Potatoes are at their best — and they preserve the most food value — when they are cooked with the skin on. Scrub, rinse them under the tap, and cook them, unpeeled, in steam or in a small amount of salted water.

For baking, preheat the oven to 400 degrees, and prepare the potatoes as above. Prick the skins in several places with a fork, and either bake as is or wrapped in aluminum foil.

Stuffed potato: when the baked potato is done, cut an X in the skin and scoop out the inside. Mash the potato with some milk, salt, and pepper until smooth (⅓ cup = 1 Bread Exchange). Garnish with parsley or paprika, or even with chives, dill, parsley, or thyme. Spoon the potato mixture back into the "jacket" and reheat briefly.

For genuine stuffing, prepare the potatoes as described and add some grated cheese (¼ cup = 1 oz meat), mushrooms, or cooked meat (ham, chicken, etc.).

To reduce cooking time to 45 minutes, cut the potato in half, and place it, sliced side down, in a lightly greased oven dish.

As a variation on boiled potatoes, substitute consommé or defatted bouillon for water; this adds new flavor and color.

Potato salad is especially good as a summer dish. To prepare, dice a cooked, cold potato (⅓ cup = 1 Bread Exchange). Mix in some mayonnaise (½ tablespoon = 1 Fat Exchange), and season to taste with chives, salt, pepper, parsley, onion, garlic, etc. Serve very cold on a bed of lettuce.

Boiled potatoes are a standard accompaniment for any main dish, such as stew or beef with vegetables, etc.
As a final suggestion, here's a good way to turn leftover mashed potatoes into Potato Cakes.

For each serving, mix ⅓ cup mashed potatoes with 1 tablespoon flour. Roll this out on a board with a rolling pin, and divide into squares. Cook each square in a very hot, oiled frying pan, or in the oven. One portion = 1½ Bread Exchanges. If the cakes are eaten with butter, 1 teaspoon = 1 Fat Exchange.

We hope some of these ideas will help vary your daily menu.

Potato Stuffing

Ingredients	**Cooked, peeled potato, mashed smooth (no fat or milk added). Season with onion salt, thyme, sage, savory, salt, and pepper.**
Preparation	Use as a stuffing for roast chicken or turkey.
Exchange Value	1 No. 8 ice cream scoop, or ⅓ cup = 1 Bread Exchange.

Potato Salad

Ingredients	**Boiled potatoes** — 2 small
	Minced onion — 2 teaspoons
	Minced celery — 1 tablespoon
	Green pepper, chopped fine — 2 teaspoons
	Chopped red pepper — optional
	Salt and pepper — optional
	Zero mayonnaise (see recipe in chapter on sauces) — 1 tablespoon
	— or —
	regular mayonnaise — 2 teaspoons for 1 Fat Exchange
	Prepared mustard — 2 teaspoons
Preparation	Dice the boiled potatoes while they're still warm. Add all the other ingredients, chill, and divide into 2 portions.
Exchange Value	1 portion = 1 Bread Exchange (with Zero mayonnaise) or 1 Bread Exchange + 1 Fat Exchange (with regular mayonnaise).
Variations	Substitute shallots for onions. Add a chopped hard-boiled egg (increase value by ½ Meat Exchange per portion). This recipe is easily increased or divided for any number of portions.

Gypsy Potatoes

Ingredients		
	Water	1½ cups
	Salt	½ teaspoon
	Butter or margarine	4 teaspoons
	Creamed cottage cheese	½ cup
	Skim milk	¼ cup
	Instant potato flakes	1 package of 3½ oz
	Poppy seeds	½ teaspoon

Preparation

Combine the water, salt, and butter in a saucepan and bring to a boil.

Use an electric mixer to blend the cottage cheese and skim milk; pour this mixture into the saucepan.

Add the potato flakes, beat well, and sprinkle with the poppy seeds.

Portions

4 half-cup servings

Exchange Value

1 portion = 1 Bread Exchange + 1 Fat Exchange + ½ Meat Exchange.

Variations

Substitute chives for the poppy seeds.

Potatoes Rose-Marie

Ingredients		
	Peeled potatoes	8 very small
	Onion, sliced thin	1 medium
	Rosemary	½ teaspoon
	Salt	1 teaspoon
	Salad oil	2 teaspoons

Preparation

Cook the potatoes until half done, or use canned, precooked potatoes.

Add the onion, rosemary, and salt; cook for 10 minutes, or until the onion is tender.

Drain.

Heat the oil in a frying pan, and brown the mixture.

Portions	4 servings of 2 potatoes each.	
Exchange Value	1 portion = 1 Bread Exchange + ½ Fat Exchange.	

Scalloped Potatoes

Ingredients	Raw potatoes, sliced	4 small
	Butter	2 teaspoons
	Flour	1 tablespoon
	Salt	½ teaspoon
	Pepper	1 pinch
	Milk	1 cup

Preparation
Lay the sliced potatoes in a 1½ quart casserole dish.
Melt the butter in a frying pan, blend in the flour and milk, and stir until the sauce thickens.
Pour over the potatoes, and place in a 375-degree oven.
Cook covered for 45 minutes; remove the lid and cook 30 minutes longer.

Portions 4

Exchange Value
1 portion = 1 Fat Exchange + 1 Bread Exchange
+ 1 Group A Vegetable Exchange.

Variation
Add 2 oz of grated cheese, and subtract ½ oz of meat per serving from the exchange allowed.

Preparing Rice: 34 Ways

When you've had enough of bread and potatoes . . . try your hand with rice (⅓ cup cooked rice = 1 Bread Exchange). Take your pick of the 34 different ways we've suggested below.

— Use well-seasoned meat stock to cook the rice.

— Sprinkle with paprika.

— Garnish with freeze-dried chives (found in the spice section of the supermarket; the freeze-drying process preserves the flavor well).

— Crumble crisp bacon on top (1 slice = 1 Fat Exchange); or mix with 1 teaspoon sour cream (½ Fat Exchange).
— Cover with an ounce of grated cheese, any kind. Place in a hot oven, or under the broiler for 2 minutes, until the cheese forms a golden crust.
— Mix in chopped mushrooms (sautéed in butter if you can afford a Fat Exchange; if not, heated in stock). Or, use the same procedure for water chestnuts (same exchange value).
— Add some sliced olives (1 Fat Exchange), or some chopped pepper, either sweet or hot (a small amount has negligible value).
— Garnish with chopped parsley.
— Melt one or two Fat Exchanges, and blend in some curry powder. Mix this in well with the rice. Excellent with chicken.
— Add peas, fresh, frozen, or canned (1 Vegetable Exchange or half this amount only).
— Add fresh or canned tomatoes.
— Use small, individual molds, preferably ring-shaped, to form the rice; garnish simply. Any other small mold would do.
— Flavor rice accompanying fish with 1 teaspoon lemon juice; 1 teaspoon orange juice for rice served with chicken or duck.
— Mix in finely-chopped sour pickles.
— When the rice is nearly cooked, add some dried onion flakes.
— Mix in grated carrot (1 small carrot = ½ Vegetable Exchange).
— Flavor with a few drops of hot steak sauce, particularly when serving with beef.
— A spoonful of apple juice with cinnamon or nutmeg added gives zest to rice served with pork.
— Substitute cranberry juice for apple juice.

If you would rather use your portion of rice in a dessert dish, try any of the menu ideas below. Often it's more convenient to prepare one cup of rice (i.e. 3 Bread Exchanges), and divide this into 3 equal dessert portions. These are suggestions for making a rice dessert special without using up too many exchanges.

— Mix cold rice with small pieces of fruit — any kind tastes good. Exchange Value = 1 Bread Exchange + 1 Fruit Exchange. Use your own canned sugarless fruit (see procedure in the preceding chapter), or the regular variety, rinsed in a colander. Frozen unsweetened fruit is available and quite suitable too, as is fresh fruit. A mixture of strawberries and melon is delicious.

— Simply flavor the rice with the syrup from a can of unsweetened fruit. In this case the Exchange Value = the amount of rice used.

— Add small pieces of orange, or grated orange peel. For something especially appealing to children, add food coloring and prepare in a mold.

— Flavor the rice with any fruit essence, available in specialized food stores.

— Add a small amount of maple extract.

— Mix in one finely-chopped date (= ½ Fruit Exchange).

— Top molded rice with meringue. To prepare, beat one egg white until stiff, adding sugar substitute, a pinch of cream of tartar, and food coloring if you wish. Brown briefly in the oven. Individual molds in different shapes — animals, etc. — are favorites with children.

— An unsweetened applesauce with some nutmeg or cinnamon; top with meringue, prepared as above. Exchange value = rice + applesauce. Since one egg is enough for 2 to 3 portions of meringue, the value of the meringue is negligible.

— Add an egg, beaten with a small amount of water and sweetened with some sugar substitute, to the warm rice; brown a few minutes in the oven. Add 1 Meat Exchange to the value of the rice.

— Rice pudding can be topped with 2 spoons of cream = 1 Fat Exchange).

Although rice is perhaps the most flexible food in the starch category, pasta can also be prepared and enjoyed many different ways.

Desserts

Baking Powder Biscuits

Ingredients		
All-purpose flour		2 cups
Baking powder		3 teaspoons
Salt		1 teaspoon
Shortening		4 tablespoons
Skim milk		¾ cup

Preparation

Sift the flour and salt together, and cut the shortening into it with a pastry blender or 2 knives.
Add the milk, stir, and knead the dough several times.
On a lightly floured board, roll the dough to a ½" thickness.
Using all the dough, cut out 15 circles of the same size.
Bake in a 450-degree oven for 12 to 15 minutes.

Portions

15 biscuits

Exchange Value

1 biscuit = 1 Bread Exchange + 1 Fat Exchange.

Blueberry Muffins

Ingredients		
Milk		1 cup
Butter		5 tablespoons
liquid sugar substitute equivalent to		⅓ cup sugar
Eggs		2
Flour		3 cups
Baking powder		5 teaspoons
Salt		⅔ teaspoon
Blueberries		1 cup

Preparation

Use 1 teaspoon of butter to grease the muffin tins.
Preheat the oven to 375 degrees.
Dredge the blueberries in ¼ cup flour.
Sift the rest of the flour with the salt and baking powder.
Cream the rest of the butter.
Beat the eggs in a separate bowl.
Add the milk and sugar substitute to the eggs.

Stir the dry and liquid ingredients alternately into the creamed butter.
Add the blueberries and stir gently.
Drop into 18 muffin tins, and bake for 25 minutes.

Portions 18 muffins

Exchange Value 1 muffin = 1 Bread Exchange + 1 Fat Exchange.

Bran Muffins

Ingredients

Milk	½ cup
Baking soda	1½ teaspoons
All Bran cereal	1½ cups
Eggs	2
Salad oil	½ cup
Sugar substitute	
All-purpose flour	1½ cups
Baking powder	½ teaspoon
Salt	1 teaspoon
Vanilla	½ teaspoon
Unsweetened applesauce	1½ cups

Preparation Combine the All Bran, milk, and baking soda, and set aside for ten minutes.
Add the eggs, salad oil, and the sugar substitute, if it is liquid.
If the sugar substitute is dry, sift with the dry ingredients.
Gradually stir the dry ingredients into the first mixture.
Flavor with vanilla, and add the applesauce.
The batter will fill 26 muffin tins; bake for 15 minutes in a 400-degree oven.

Portions 26

Exchange Value 1 muffin = 1 Bread Exchange + 1 Fat Exchange.

130

Bread Pudding

Ingredients		
	Breadcrumbs	1 slice
	Apple, peeled and sliced thin, or	1 small
	Seedless raisins	1½ tablespoons, steamed
	Skim milk	2 tablespoons
	Egg, beaten	1
	Sugar substitute	optional

Preparation
If the bread is stale, pour boiling water over it and let drain.
Place the bread and the sliced apple or raisins in a baking dish.
Add the beaten egg, milk, and sugar substitute, and brown in
a 350-degree oven.

Portions   2

Exchange Value
1 portion = 1 Bread Exchange + ½ Meat Exchange.

Chocolate Brownies

Ingredients		
	Butter or margarine	½ cup
	Sugar substitute equivalent to	¼ cup sugar
	Unsweetened chocolate	2 squares
	Eggs	2
	Vanilla	½ teaspoon
	All-purpose flour	¾ cup
	Double action baking powder	1 teaspoon
	Chopped nuts	½ cup

Preparation
Preheat the oven to 350 degrees.
Cream the butter with the sugar substitute.
Add the melted chocolate, and beat the mixture till smooth.
Mix in the eggs and vanilla.
Add the flour, baking powder, and nuts, and beat till creamy.
Pour into a buttered pan, 8" x 8" x 2".
Bake for 30 minutes, or until the top is glossy.
Leave in the pan to cool.

Divide into 16 portions.

**Exchange
Value**

1 portion = ½ Bread Exchange + 2 Fat Exchanges.

Oatmeal Cookies

Ingredients		
Soft margarine		**½ cup**
Liquid sugar substitute		**4 teaspoons**
Vanilla		**1 teaspoon**
Egg		**1**
Cold water		**¾ cup**
All-purpose flour		**1 cup**
Salt		**½ teaspoon**
Baking soda		**½ teaspoon**
Cinnamon		**1 teaspoon**
Instant rolled oats		**1 cup**
Raisins		**½ cup**

Preparation

Combine the margarine, sugar substitute, vanilla, and the egg in a large bowl.
Beat with an electric mixer, at high speed, for 2 minutes.
Add the water, flour, salt, soda, cinnamon, and beat at slow speed for another 2 minutes.
Mix in the rolled oats and raisins.
Drop from a teaspoon onto an ungreased cookie sheet.
Bake in a 375-degree oven, for 12 to 15 minutes.

Portions

42 cookies

**Exchange
Value**

1 cookie = ½ Group B Vegetable Exchange + ½ Fat Exchange.
2 cookies = 1 Fruit Exchange + 1 Fat Exchange.

Orange Bran Cookies

Ingredients	All-purpose flour	2 cups
	Baking powder	1 teaspoon
	Salt	¼ teaspoon
	Bran Flakes	1 cup
	Soft butter, or margarine	½ cup
	Egg	1
	Unsweetened orange juice	2 tablespoons
	Grated orange peel	1 teaspoon
	Lemon extract	½ teaspoon
	Sugar substitute equivalent to	2 cups sugar

Preparation

Sift together the first 3 ingredients.
Add the rest of the ingredients, and mix into a dough.
Form the dough into 2 half-inch thick rolls. Wrap in aluminum foil.
Chill several hours, or overnight.

Portions

Cut into 44 slices of equal thickness. Place on a lightly greased cookie sheet, and bake in a 400-degree oven for 8 to 12 minutes.

Exchange Value

2 cookies = 1 Fruit Exchange or 1 Group B Vegetable Exchange
+ 1 Fat Exchange.

Orange Chiffon Cake

Ingredients	Egg whites	8
	Sifted flour	2¼ cups
	Salt	1 teaspoon
	Whole egg yolks	5
	Double action baking powder	3 teaspoons
	Orange peel, grated	3 tablespoons
	Sugar substitute equivalent to 1½ cups sugar plus enough orange juice to make	¾ cup
	Cream of tartar	½ teaspoon
	Salad oil	½ cup

133

Preparation **At least 3 hours before serving time:**
a)   Separate the eggs, putting whites in a large bowl and yolks in a small one. Let them reach room temperature.
b)   In a large bowl, sift together the flour, salt, and baking powder. Grate the orange peel and combine the sugar substitute with the orange juice for later use.

When you are ready to cook:
c)   Preheat the oven to 325 degrees. Rinse a square 9" cake pan with cold water, and drain.
d)   Add the cream of tartar to the egg whites, and beat until they are very stiff, past the "peaked" stage for making meringues.
e)   Make a well in the middle of the dry ingredients, and add the salad oil, orange peel, and orange juice and sugar substitute mixture. Mix them well, and beat with an electric mixer, medium speed, for 1 minute.
.f)   Gently combine this mixture with the beaten egg whites, folding in until completely mixed. Carefully pour into the cake pan, and bake 35 minutes until golden yellow.
g)   Cool for 20 minutes; run a knife around the edge of the cake, and gently lift with fingers to detach from bottom of the pan. Turn upside down on a cake rack to cool.

Portions   16

Exchange Value   1 portion = ½ Meat Exchange + 1 Bread Exchange + 1 Fat Exchange.

Peanut Butter Cookies

Ingredients		
All-purpose flour	1¼ cups
Liquid sugar substitute	1 tablespoon
Baking powder	1½ teaspoons
Vanilla	1 teaspoon
Homogenized peanut butter	½ cup
Salad oil	¼ cup
Water	¼ cup
Egg	1

Preparation	Combine all the ingredients in a large bowl. Drop by teaspoonsful onto an ungreased cookie sheet.
	Press the cookies flat with a fork.
	Bake in a 375-degree oven for 12 to 15 minutes.

Portions	42 cookies

Exchange Value	1 cookie = ½ Group B Vegetable Exchange + ½ Fat Exchange.
	2 cookies = 1 Fruit Exchange + 1 Fat Exchange.

Pie Crust

Ingredients	All-purpose flour	1 cup
	Butter, margarine, shortening, or vegetable oil	¼ cup or 4 tablespoons
	Ice water	⅓ cup or less

Preparation	Cut the shortening or butter into the flour with a pastry blender or 2 knives.
	Quickly moisten with the ice water, form the dough into a ball, and refrigerate.

Exchange Value	The whole recipe = 8 Bread Exchanges + 12 Fat Exchanges.

Variations	If you use all the dough for 1 pie crust, and the pie is cut into 8 equal slices, each slice = 1 Bread Exchange + 1½ Fat Exchanges.
	If the dough is divided into 4 parts to make individual pies, the value of each = 2 Bread Exchanges + 3 Fat Exchanges.
	If the dough is divided into 8, for making tarts, the value of each = 1 Bread Exchange + 1½ Fat Exchanges.

Popovers

Ingredients		
	Eggs	2
	Skim milk	1 cup
	All-purpose flour	1 cup
	Salt	¼ teaspoon
	Butter or margarine	1 tablespoon

Preparation Beat the eggs, and add the milk.
Sift together the flour and salt, and gradually add to the eggs and milk.
Beat until creamy.
Add the melted butter or margarine.
Pour into 8 lightly greased deep muffin tins, or custard cups.
Bake in a 425-degree oven for 40 minutes.

Portions 8 popovers

Exchange Value 1 portion = 1 Bread Exchange + ½ Fat Exchange.

Special Macaroons

Ingredients		
	Egg white, well beaten	1
	Liquid sugar substitute	½ teaspoon
	Almond extract	⅛ teaspoon
	Corn flakes	1 cup

Preparation Beat the egg white until stiff, and add the sugar substitute and almond extract.
Stir in the corn flakes, and use a teaspoon to drop onto an ungreased cookie sheet.
Bake for 10 minutes in a 375-degree oven.

Portions 12

Exchange Value 5 macaroons = 1 Bread Exchange.

Sponge Cake

Ingredients		
Eggs, separated		**5**
All-purpose flour		**1 cup**
Sugar		**½ cup**
Sugar substitute		**1 teaspoon + 1 table-spoon water**
Cream of tartar		**¼ teaspoon**
Salt		**¼ teaspoon**
Lemon juice		**1 tablespoon**

Preparation Beat the egg whites, salt, and cream of tartar until peaks will form, adding in the sugar as you beat.
In another bowl, beat together the yolks, sugar substitute, and lemon juice.
Stir the yolk mixture into the egg whites.
Pour into a 9″ ungreased angel cake pan, and bake for 45 minutes in a 350-degree oven.

Portions Divide into 10 equal pieces.

Exchange Value 1 slice = 1 Bread Exchange + ½ Fat Exchange + ½ Fruit Exchange.

Variation Serve with a ½ Fruit Exchange of fresh or frozen, unsweetened small fruits, such as strawberries, raspberries, or blueberries.

Strawberry Pie

Ingredients	Corn flakes, crushed	¾ cup (or 2¼ cups uncrushed)
	Margarine	3 tablespoons
	Sugar substitute equivalent to	1 tablespoon sugar
Fillings	Thawed and drained frozen strawberries, unsweetened (reserve the juice)	2 cups
	Add water to the juice to make	⅔ cup
	Unsweetened strawberry gelatin	1 envelope
	Lemon juice	⅓ cup
	Egg whites	2
	Sugar substitute equivalent to	½ cup sugar (optional)

Preparation

Crust

Preheat the oven to 375 degrees.
Mix together the first 3 ingredients, and use the back of a spoon to press into a lining for a 9" pie plate.
Bake for 8 minutes and let cool.

Filling

Combine the juice, water, and gelatin in a small saucepan.
Heat, stirring constantly, until the gelatin is dissolved.
Add the lemon juice and sugar substitute.
Refrigerate until the mixture has thickened to the consistency of an egg white.
Add the 2 egg whites, and beat at top speed until light and frothy.
Add the drained strawberries.
Pour into the pie crust, and refrigerate at least 3 hours before serving.

Portions

Divide into 8 sections.

Exchange Value

1 portion = 1 Bread Exchange + 1 Fat Exchange.

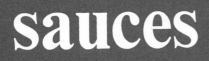

sauces

Sauces and Salad Dressings

Sauces

It takes a few culinary tricks to prepare a sauce that conforms to the restrictions of your diet, since this is a "luxury" item on the menu.

First of all, learn the composition of the 3 kinds of sauces that are basic to a good menu.

A. Sauces to Accompany Meat or Vegetables
— Made from a bouillon or milk base.
— The thickening agent is usually flour. The proportion is 1 tablespoon (½ Bread Exchange) to one cup liquid for a light sauce; 2 tablespoons (1 Bread Exchange) for a thicker sauce.
— Enriched with butter, margarine, or animal fat (whatever exchanges are allowed).
— Salt, pepper, and other seasonings are used to enhance the flavor. Choice of seasoning is very important.

B. Dressings for Salads
— Based on oil and vinegar, or simply on vinegar, or lemon juice.
— seasoned with salt, pepper, and other spices.

C. Sauces to accompany Fruits
— Based on fruit juices, or carbonated diet drinks.
— A thickening agent other than flour, such as:
  Cornstarch — 2 tablespoons = 1 Bread Exchange.
  Tapioca — 1 teaspoon (negligible value) has a thickening power = 1 tablespoon flour.

White Sauce

Ingredients		
	Butter	2 teaspoons
	Flour	2 tablespoons
	Skim milk, warm	1 cup
	Salt and pepper and seasonings	to taste

Preparation

Melt the butter over low heat.
Blend the flour into the butter with a wooden spoon; do not let it brown.
Gradually add the warm milk, stirring constantly until the sauce thickens.
When the sauce has reached the desired thickness, add the seasonings and continue cooking for 10 to 15 minutes, depending on the amount of flour used and the heat.

Portions

2 half-cup servings

Exchange Value

1 portion = ½ Milk Exchange + ½ Bread Exchange.

Variations

If whole milk is used, the value increases by 2 Fat Exchanges.
Vegetables, Group A or B, can be added to the sauce; as well as meat, eggs, cheese, or fish, depending on the exchanges available.

Salad Dressing

Ingredients		
	Tomato juice	1 cup
	Lemon juice	¼ cup
	Onion	2 tablespoons
	Salt, pepper, green pepper, parsley, dried mustard	to taste

Preparation

Combine the ingredients in a jar with a screw-top lid.
Refrigerate, and shake well before using.

Exchange Value

None

French Dressing

Ingredients		
	Tomato juice	1 cup
	Grapefruit juice, unsweetened	½ cup
	Bouillon or consommé	½ cup
	Garlic powder	⅛ teaspoon
	Salt and pepper	to taste

Preparation Combine all the ingredients in a jar or bottle, shake well; chill, with the lid on, for at least half an hour.

Portions 2 cups

Exchange Value Negligible, for a 2-tablespoon serving.

Tomato Sauce

Ingredients		
	Vegetable oil	1 tablespoon
	Minced onion	1 medium
	Minced garlic	1 clove
	Canned tomatoes	28 oz
	Bay leaf	1
	Chopped parsley	2 tablespoons
	Oregano	to taste
	Salt	½ teaspoon
	Pepper	⅛ teaspoon
	Liquid sugar substitute	a few drops

Preparation Cook the onion and garlic in the hot oil until they are tender, but not browned.
Add the tomatoes, bay leaf, parsley, oregano, salt, and pepper.
Cover and simmer very gently for about an hour, stirring occasionally.
Just before serving, add the sugar substitute.

Portions Divide into 6 equal helpings.

Exchange Value 1 portion (½ cup) = negligible.

Spaghetti Sauce

Ingredients		
Tomato juice		2 cups
Tomato paste		1 teaspoon
Cornstarch		2 tablespoons
Dry mustard		1 teaspoon
Vinegar		4 tablespoons
Thyme, parsley, pepper, salt		to taste

Preparation

Mix together the cornstarch, mustard, and seasonings.
Use a bit of cold water to make this into a paste.
Bring the tomato juice, tomato paste, and vinegar to a boil.
Add the cornstarch mixture to this, and cook over low heat.

Exchange Value

½ cup sauce = 1 Group A Vegetable Exchange.
1 cup sauce = 1 Group B Vegetable Exchange
+ ½ Bread Exchange.

Variation

Add meatballs, made from lean meat, (1 oz, or 1 Meat Exchange according to the calculations of your own diet).
Cook the meatballs over very low heat, let cool, and drain off the fat.

Note

This recipe can be frozen and used any time.

Curry Sauce

Ingredients		
Canned tomatoes		28 oz
or		
Tomato juice		28 oz
Salt		1 teaspoon
Dried onion flakes		1 teaspoon
Curry powder		1 teaspoon
Pepper		¼ teaspoon
Dry breadcrumbs		¼ cup

Preparation

Combine all the ingredients in a saucepan, and simmer 15 minutes.

Exchange Value

½ cup = 1 Group A Vegetable Exchange.

Hot Sauce

Ingredients	Cornstarch	1½ tablespoons
	Salt	¼ teaspoon
	Cinnamon	¼ teaspoon
	Lime Carbonated drink, low-calorie	8 oz (1 cup)

Preparation Combine the cornstarch, salt, and cinnamon in a saucepan.
Blend smooth with about 1 tablespoon of lime drink.
Gradually stir in the rest of the drink and cook over low heat,
until the mixture is clear and thick.

Exchange Negligible, in small amounts.

Variations Use the sauce as a topping for baked apple; or add a small amount
of sugar substitute and serve over a piece of plain cake, or with
biscuits.
Prepare with low-calorie ginger ale, flavor with mint, and serve
over a pear.

Brown Sauce

Ingredients	Flour, browned	1 tablespoon
	Beef consommé	¾ cup
	Lemon juice	
	Parsley	

Preparation Heat the consommé.
Blend the flour into a paste with a bit of cold water.
Add this to the boiling consommé, and stir until thick.
Cook over low heat for about 10 minutes.
Flavor with lemon juice and parsley.

Exchange Value None, if portions are limited to about ¼ cup.

Variation Substitute chicken stock for the beef consommé.

Fruit Sauce

Ingredients	Unsweetened orange juice	1 cup
	Lemon juice	6 tablespoons
	Paprika	¼ teaspoon
	Nutmeg or cinnamon	

Preparation Combine all the ingredients in a jar or bottle with a lid, and chill at least half an hour.
Shake before serving.

Quantity 1½ cups

Exchange Value 2 tablespoons = negligible

Barbecue Sauce

Ingredients	Onion, finely chopped	¼ cup
	Catsup	1 cup
	Water	½ cup
	Lemon juice	¼ cup
	Worcestershire sauce	2 teaspoons
	Vinegar	2 teaspoons
	Dry mustard	½ teaspoon
	Sugar substitute	1 teaspoon

Preparation Combine everything in a saucepan and simmer for about 20 minutes.

Exchange Value ½ cup portion = 1 Group A Vegetable Exchange.
¼ cup portion = negligible

Sour Cream Sauce

Ingredients	Plain yogurt	6 oz
	Lemon juice	3 tablespoons
	Prepared mustard	¼ teaspoon
	Salad oil	¼ teaspoon
	Salt	¼ teaspoon

Preparation	Combine all the ingredients in a jar with a lid, chill for at least half an hour, and shake well before using.
Quantity	1 cup
Exchange Value	1 tablespoon portion = negligible

Garlic Sauce

Ingredients	Buttermilk	1 cup
	Garlic, pressed	1 clove
	Lemon juice	1 - 1½ teaspoons
	Dry mustard	¼ teaspoon

Preparation	Combine the buttermilk, garlic, and mustard in a jar. Add the lemon juice and shake vigorously. Chill, with the lid on, for 30 minutes.
Quantity	1 cup
Exchange Value	2 tablespoon portion = negligible

Tartar Sauce

Ingredients	Viennese Mayonnaise (see recipe in this chapter)	1 cup (amount of recipe)
	Parsley	1 tablespoon
	Chives	1 tablespoon
	Tarragon	1 tablespoon
	Capers, finely chopped	1 tablespoon
	Dill pickle, chopped	1 small slice

Preparation	Combine all the ingredients, cover, and refrigerate at least half an hour.
Exchange Value	2 tablespoons = ½ Fat Exchange.

Vinaigrette Zero

Ingredients	Tomato juice	2½ cups
	Lemon juice	5 oz
	Chopped onion	¼ cup
	Chopped parsley	½ tablespoon
	Salt and pepper	to taste

Preparation Combine all the ingredients in a screw-top jar, refrigerate with the lid on, and shake vigorously just before using.

Exchange Value 1 tablespoon = none

Party Relish

Ingredients	Green pepper, chopped	1
	Red pepper, chopped	1
	Onion	½ small
	Vinegar	1 tablespoon
	Saccharine	1 tablet

Preparation Combine everything in a saucepan, cover with salted water, and boil until the vegetables are tender.

Exchange Value 1 Group A Vegetable Exchange, or negligible in small amounts.

Zero Mayonnaise

Ingredients	Mineral oil	2½ cups
	Egg yolks	3
	Vinegar	¼ cup
	Dry mustard	¾ teaspoon
	Paprika	1 teaspoon

Preparation   Beat the egg yolks, and add the seasonings.
Add the mineral oil, by the teaspoonful at first, and when ¼ cup has been mixed in, by the tablespoonful.
Reduce the consistency by adding the vinegar.

**Exchange
Value**   1 tablespoon = none

Viennese Mayonnaise

Ingredients		
Egg yolks, hard-boiled		**2**
Raw egg yolks		**2**
Plain yogurt		**6 oz**
Lemon juice		**½ teaspoon**
Salt, white pepper		**½ teaspoon**

Preparation   Crumble the cooked egg yolks very finely, and mix into a smooth paste with the 2 raw egg yolks.
Add the other ingredients, and whisk the mixture energetically.
Cover and cool for at least 30 minutes before serving.

Portions   1 cup

**Exchange
Value**   1 teaspoon = negligible
1½ tablespoons = ½ Fat Exchange

helpful hints

Helpful Hints

Helpful Hints

What am I going to make for dinner . . ?

What should we eat today? — a familiar refrain for everyone, not just the diabetic or the person on a special diet.

Every day of our lives, at least three times a day, the routine necessity of eating in order to survive brings along with it the necessity of choosing: **what** to eat?

For some people, food is a constant source of delight and the object of careful thought and preparation. For others, eating is just a tedious chore to get out of the way. Meals are an opportunity for some to cheat on the diet; for others, it's a daily act of self-discipline.

Whatever your attitude towards food, everyone faces the same basic problems, and eventually comes to realize that eating well is an Art.

To practise any art — unless you're a born natural — first you have to acquaint yourself with the Science that corresponds to it. What do we know about nutrition? There is a number of basics to know in order to eat well.

Know what you are able to eat, and what you **ought** to eat. For everyone, whether or not they are restricted to a special diet, there are some foods that are essential to health, and others that are superfluous, or even harmful.

Know how to plan and select meals that take into consideration local or seasonal foods, budget demands, personal preferences, and above all, the needs of each individual. Plan a careful budget and stick to it when meal-planning and shopping. Too often people use the excuse that "I just can't afford to follow my diet!"

Know how to prepare and use food properly. So often fine food can be ruined by careless or heavyhanded cooking.

Besides these fundamentals, there are two other important considerations that affect how you eat.

Will you be eating at home, or in a cafeteria, restaurant, a friend's place, or perhaps outdoors, on a camping trip? It may mean you won't have to cook, but you will still have the problem of choosing what to eat.

What kind of attitude do you have to food, and what kind of atmosphere do you create for mealtimes? You don't have to serve elaborate meals to create a family dinner that is a peaceful and pleasant part of the day . . . a carefully set table, interesting conversation, and a quiet atmosphere are all important to a healthy, relaxing meal.

Adapting the calculated diet to different situations

RESTAURANTS

Yes, it's possible to eat regularly in hotels and restaurants and still stick to your prescribed diet.

First of all, explain the situation to your dietician or doctor, who will adjust your prescription, and outline the changes to you. Secondly, memorize the food substitutions that your diet permits. Thirdly, study the menus of the restaurants you usually eat in, to determine which one fits in best with your diet.

The diabetic who makes these efforts will soon realize that eating out is no longer an impossibility — in fact, it can be relatively easy, and even interesting. You'll find that if you ask, the restaurateurs may even alter the menu for you.

Soon you'll discover that although you are in a minority, you're not alone, and that waiters and other staff tend to be more sympathetic and helpful than you might anticipate. Finally, you'll be introduced to new dishes that you may not have tried before, simply out of force of habit.

So what can a diabetic expect to be able to eat in a moderately-priced restaurant?

Breakfast presents no problem. Any restaurant, large or small, can offer you fresh orange juice or tomato juice, dry toast if you specify it, eggs prepared any way your diet permits, even crisp bacon, and black coffee. You couldn't ask for anything easier to calculate; all in all, breakfast is a simpler matter eating out than at home.

Lunch is a bit more problematic, but can be solved. Below is a sample menu from a moderately-priced restaurant. The choice of permissible items will obviously be much broader in better restaurants.

MENU

Soupe du jour — Consommé
Tomato juice, apple juice
    Daily Special
Pork sausages
Hamburger steak
Chef salad
Cold roast pork
Calves' liver and bacon
Pork chops
Omelettes
Hot chicken sandwich
Sliced ham and pineapple
Chicken or Salmon Salad
Small Spencer stead, served on a board, vegetables included
    Desserts
Blancmange
Strawberry jello
Stewed prunes
Home-made vanilla or chocolate cake
Pies
    Tea, coffee

Soup: Choose the consommé, if it doesn't have too much grease in it. Either of the juices offered are equivalent to a Group A Vegetable Exchange, a Group B Vegetable Exchange, or a Fruit Exchange. The consommé has no value.

Main course: You can choose from among the hamburger (no sauce), the roast pork or pork chops (trim the fat off), the omelette, the Spencer steak, or the calves' liver, with or without the bacon.

All these meals are served with mashed or boiled potatoes, and usually a Group B Vegetable; you can also order a small salad to complete the vegetable exchange. Judge the amount of meat you are allowed by eye — this is something you should be accustomed to doing.

You can order the Chef Salad and supplement it with 2 eggs, or some cheese. Calculate the chicken or salmon salad as is, including the mayonnaise used in them. Bread and butter are optional, according to your own diet.

Jello is all right for dessert, if there's no alternative, but it's easier to bring along a piece of fruit, or use the before-lunch juice for this exchange. Tea and coffee — no problem.

In better restaurants, you can choose from a wider selection of grilled meats, salads, and vegetables. Often, sugar-free canned fruit salads are available, or whatever fresh fruit is in season; this will take care of dessert.

Diabetics who eat out will find they can enjoy a whole range of food. Just be sure to study the menu so that you can adapt it to your personal diet.

CAMPING

With camping so popular these days, diabetics may find the following recipes or cooking methods useful. These can also be prepared at home, in a medium-hot oven.

Campfire Dinner: For each person, place the ingredients below in a 10″ square piece of aluminum foil, either doubled, or the thick type:

    Chopped meat (whatever your own exchange should be)
    Raw carrots, sliced thin (½ cup, or 2 medium carrots)
    1 medium potato, sliced thin
    1 slice of raw onion
    1 tablespoon water
    salt and pepper

Fold the aluminum foil into a tightly-sealed envelope, and cook on a grill, or right amongst the glowing coals if your fire isn't too high. In 20 minutes you'll have a superb dinner.

Exchange Value: 1 Bread Exchange + 1 Group B Vegetable Exchange + 2 or 3 Meat Exchanges.

Baked Apple: Lightly butter a 10" square piece of thick aluminum foil. Fill the centre of a cored, medium-sized apple with 1 teaspoon raisins, 2 tablespoons water, and some sugar substitute (optional). Close the foil around the apple, seal it well, and bake the same as the dinner above, for half an hour. Dessert will be ready and waiting when the main course is over.

Exchange Value: 1 Fruit Exchange + 1 Group A Vegetable Exchange, or
2 Group A Vegetable Exchanges, or
1½ Fruit Exchanges.

Shish-ke-bab:
Sprinkle 1"-square cubes of meat (the appropriate exchanges according to your diet) with meat tenderizer and garlic salt. Cut a medium onion into ½" slices. Cut two small tomatoes, or one medium, in half. Spear the meat, onion, and tomatoes alternately on a metal skewer, or a green branch. Cook slowly, turning it over the fire, for 15 to 20 minutes.

Exchange Value: Meat + Group A + Group B Vegetables.

PICNICS

Nice weather means vacation time, outings, and trips to the countryside for some long-awaited outdoor recreation at the end of winter.

Diabetics, used to being restricted by the demands of their diet, may consider picnics just another food problem to solve. But there's no reason to be excluded from Sunday picnics, or even extended wilderness holidays. The diabetic's régime is so simple and basically sensible, that with a little foresight you should be able to cope with every situation that an active, changing life includes. Let's consider a few possibilities.

Charlie owns a cottage where he spends every weekend and his vacation. Dealing with his diet is no problem for him, since he stocks up on provisions in the city before leaving. He always remembers to bring along a supply of special fruit, which may be unavailable in smaller towns. He would also be smart to include some low-calorie juices and drinks, to eliminate the temptation of sweetened juices, carbonated pop, and other prohibited items.

For Mrs. Johnson, a recent diabetic, the situation is different. On Sundays, her family likes to get together outdoors for a picnic dinner. Rather than depriving her family or herself of this weekly pleasure, she can enjoy a genuine picnic meal like the one described below.

> Tomato juice (= 1 Vegetable Exchange)
> Sandwiches: 4 slices of sandwich bread, crusts removed
>   = 2 Bread Exchanges
> 3 oz of lean ham
> 1 pat of butter
> Lettuce
> Mustard (optional)
> Celery sticks
> 1 small raw carrot (grated or sliced in strips)
> Dessert: ½ cantaloupe, or 1 small apple
> Iced tea with a slice of lemon

Sheila's son is a teenager who would rather eat in places like drive-in restaurants. The menus tend to be all the same, without much variety.

Hamburger: the roll = 2 Bread Exchanges, or 1 Bread Exchange + 2 Vegetable Exchanges. Usually the pattie = 3 oz meat; although some places use 4 oz, and cheaper hamburgers can be 2 oz. Butter, mustard, and relish is sometimes included.

If his diet allows another exchange of bread and butter, a side-order of french fries (half-cup, or 6 to 10 fries) can be added. He can take along a piece of fresh fruit as dessert. Unsweetened orange is usually available most places, for a value of 1 Fruit Exchange, or 1 Group B Vegetable Exchange.

Jeannette is only nine years old, and a diabetic; but this doesn't have to interfere with picnic lunches in the park with her friends.

Have on hand some cold, bottled mineral water to take along instead of carbonated soft drinks, or give her a thermos of juice made from no-calorie concentrate (sold in the special-food sections of large supermarkets). This concentrate can also be frozen in molds with sticks, to make tasty, home-made popsicles. Prepare the picnic sandwiches described earlier, varying them if you want to by substituting a slice of non-fatty cheese, or a chopped hard-boiled egg for the meat portion. Substitute a bag of potato chips (15 large chips) for bread and butter. For dessert, fresh fruit.

And last of all, we have Mr. LaRue, self-styled gourmet, who performs as chef in his own backyard when he entertains guests. His barbecue meal is well-balanced:

> Beef consommé
> 3-oz steak, cooked in the barbecue grill
> Potato wrapped in foil and buried in the coals
> Half a hamburger bun, spread with half a pat of butter
> Salad: half portion of tomato and half a portion of cucumber
>> 1 portion green peas
>> Chopped lettuce and celery
>> Vinegar, or Zero mayonnaise (see Sauces chapter),
>> and seasonings
> Dessert: Diet jello with half a banana, or a half cup of canned
>> diet fruit salad
> Black coffee

These suggestions should be just a beginning; try experimenting with all the substitutes permitted in your diet, and you'll discover your own favorite combinations.

Diabetics can enjoy any holiday without jeopardizing their health by planning meals that could easily double as ordinary, hot-weather fare for anyone.

SUMMER MEALS

Summer Fruits and Vegetables: This is the time of year when you ought to take advantage of the low price and abundance of garden-fresh fruit and vegetables; they'll be cheaper than the canned product, or year-round items. Why not try something new — a different melon, or romaine, or escarole instead of iceberg lettuce.

159

Cheeses: These are a good substitute for meat in hot weather. Cheese has all the requirements for a main dish, and in the large markets you can take your pick from among 80 or more varieties.

Fresh Fish: If there's somebody who fishes in your family, you're in luck. Otherwise, shop for fresh fish in the market, or use canned fish. You'll find it a welcome change of pace from meat, served with fresh vegetables.

Fresh Fruit Desserts: Easy to make with diet gelatin and fresh fruit, or sugar-free, home-canned fruit. Try a fruit mousse: one well beaten fresh egg white will produce enough for 4 servings. In this case, you only need to count the value of the fruit used. Remember that berries keep well in the refrigerator. Place them in a glass bowl with a bit of powdered or liquid sugar substitute, and cover with Saran Wrap.

Meats: Have you investigated the range of canned meats at your supermarket? Add to your list of meat exchanges ready-to-use items such as whole canned chickens, or boned, jellied chicken, corned beef, pickled tongue.

When you're preparing a picnic, some small touches can make a big difference to sandwiches. A spoonful of grated raw carrot with chicken, a pinch of dry mustard mixed with chopped ham, or a bit of onion juice in egg salad sandwiches will brighten up the flavors. Don't forget to add sour pickles, sliced or chopped, or dill pickles served whole.

Beverages: Iced tea with lemon is always popular. You might try one of the new sugarless powdered mixes; in any case, a mint leaf finishes it off nicely. Iced coffee is good too!

Two lemons = 1 Fruit Exchange. Squeezing the juice and then boiling the peels makes a good lemonade. When the water cools, add the juice. Limes can also be used.

And finally, more and more low-calorie drinks are becoming commercially available. Check with your doctor or dietician to see which you can include in your diet. One of these sugar-free drinks comes in the form of an effervescent tablet; all you have to do is keep a container of iced water on hand for a cold, delicious drink in any flavor you like — one of the practical, low-cost, and varied ways to quench your thirst!

LUNCHES TO TAKE TO SCHOOL

If a school-age child has a good breakfast and a solid supper, lunch doesn't have to be a big amount. Nevertheless, it should include these five elements:

1. A source of carbohydrates: bread, rolls, a hot dog or hamburger bun, pasta, potatoes, rice, soda crackers, or some other type of cracker, muffins, a small piece of cake.

2. A source of protein. Meat, eggs, fish, cheese, sauce or soup made with meat or milk, peanut butter.

3. A vegetable: Something raw to nibble on, or in a salad or sandwich.
   Cooked, in soup, or a thermos meal.
   If a vegetable is omitted, pack an extra fruit.

4. A fruit: Raw — for dessert or snack.
   Cooked — in a dessert, or the canned diet variety.

5. Milk or beverage: Milk isn't an imperative if your son or daughter gets enough to drink at home; also, it's not always available cold at school. Include milk in the diet by using it in soups or desserts. For something to drink with school lunches, provide fruit juices, mixed vegetable juices (V8), or tomato juice. Low-calorie soft drinks are acceptable too, although they have no nutritional value.

Useful Equipment

1. A small bottle with a wide mouth. The top of the thermos doubles as a mug, and this way you can supply your child with a variety of hot meals that are easy to eat.

2. A small, wide-mouthed thermos bottle made of plastic or styrofoam, available at the larger stores. These are ideal for cold foods — puddings, salads, etc. Fill the thermos on the preceding day and refrigerate overnight; it will still be good and cold at lunchtime.

161

3. Saran Wrap. Useful for wrapping everything from sandwiches to carrot sticks.

4. Small glass jars (baby-food kind), with secure lids, for desserts. Tight closing bottles for juices.

5. Various small plastic containers (yogurt or cottage cheese cartons), or plastic-coated cartons that won't absorb flavors. Pack salads or vegetables in these.

6. Plastic sandwich bags. Some of these are sturdy enough to use again and again, and they come with a strip or flap that does a better job of sealing than the ordinary bags.

7. A Teflon-coated saucepan, for quick reheating of hot meals in the morning. Let your son or daughter take care of this.

8. Hopefully, salt, pepper, and bottle-opener are available to all the students at school. Otherwise these tend to go astray in the process of being carted back and forth from home to school.

Tricks and Timesavers

1. There are plenty of hot meals that can be made ahead of time and reheated in the morning. A number of recipes freeze well in individual portions. Some of the meals that are popular with schoolchildren:
   — Spaghetti and meatballs
   — Stew with meatballs and chunks of potato
   — Beef or chicken hash
   — Beef with vegetables, or chicken with vegetables, in a special sauce (see Sauces chapter)
   — Creamed eggs, salmon, or tuna
   — Cream soups
   — Macaroni and cheese
   — Wieners and beans

2. Buttered slices of white or brown bread, without filling, stay fresher than a sandwich, and children like to eat them along with a slice of chicken, a chicken leg, a hard-boiled egg, or a piece of cheese.

3. Leave the butter out of the refrigerator so that it's easy to spread in the morning, or use soft margarine. It's always a better

idea to put mayonnaise or mustard between 2 slices of meat, or between the lettuce and the meat; spread on the bread and left in a lunchbox at room temperature, the sandwich has a tendency to become unappetizingly soggy. You can hardly ever go wrong with peanut butter sandwiches, and they keep well. For easier eating, remember to cut the sandwiches at home, varying the size and shape. If your child is old enough to have mastered opening a tin of sardines, this makes a popular lunch accompanied with a buttered roll.

4. Vegetables stay crisp in Saran Wrap, or sealed Baggies: sticks of celery, carrot, or cucumber, shallots, radishes, sections of lettuce or tomatoes, pickles, olives, cherry tomatoes.
Salads: cole slaw doesn't lose its flavor, even left at room temperature. Pack potato salad, with or without eggs, chicken, or salmon salad in the cold thermos, with lettuce. Or, chef salad with individually-wrapped sections of Gruyère cheese, or carrot and raisin salad.

5. Fruits: The apple, an all-time favorite; oranges, or easy-to-peel mandarins; grapes, freshly packed in a plastic container so they won't be crushed; bananas — not too ripe, for they can easily become too soft sitting in a lunchbox. Cold baked apple, or canned fruit can be carried in a glass jar or plastic container with a lid, or in the cold thermos. Puddings made from milk, rice, or bread can be kept well the same way. A peeled orange will stay moist wrapped in Saran.

6. You can prepare sandwich fillings the day before, so that your son or daughter can make up the sandwich in the morning. Don't add mayonnaise or dressing ahead of time. In hot weather, use small plastic or waxed containers (1-oz size) with lids, for carrying catsup, mayonnaise, salad dressing, mustard, relish, etc.

7. It's a good idea to provide a hot meal for lunch as often as you can, and to avoid the monotony of sandwiches every single day. Surprises can also do a lot for the appetite, and the spirits.

8. Age is important. For a six- or seven-year-old, it's difficult to handle more than a schoolbag; and a hot thermos can easily be dropped and broken.

Sample Menus

For six- to nine-year-olds

Sliced chicken
Buttered rolls
Celery and carrot sticks
Mandarin orange
Milk

Hard-boiled eggs
Pickles and olives
Buttered hot dog roll
Canned fruit
Milk

Tomato juice
Sections of Gruyère cheese
Ritz crackers
Celery
Rice pudding

Vegetable soup
Cheddar or Camembert cheese
Dry biscuits and canned fruit
Milk

Peanut butter sandwich
Fresh fruit
Milk

Cheese sandwich (any kind)
Shallots
Cucumber
Mandarin or plain orange
Milk

Cream of tomato soup
Chicken salad on lettuce
Buttered Melba toast
Banana

Cocktail sausages in hot tomato
  sauce
Buttered brown bread
Special muffin (see Starchy Foods
  chapter)
Fruit juice

Creamed eggs with potatoes
Carrot sticks
Grapes
Milk

Tomato juice
Ham sandwich
Green salad
Apple
Milk

Chicken sandwich
Carrot and raisin salad
Oatmeal cookies
Fruit juice

Beef with vegetables
Buttered rolls
Tomato
Orange
Milk

Wieners and beans
Lettuce
Unsweetened pickles
Buttered bread
Canned, unsweetened pineapple
Milk

For 9-year-olds and over

Cream of chicken soup
Sections of Gruyère cheese
Soda crackers
Celery sticks
Mandarin orange
Milk

Sliced chicken or chicken leg
Buttered French bread
Cole slaw
Canned or fresh fruit
Milk

Spaghetti and meatballs
Lettuce, chopped and seasoned
Unsweetened fruit salad
Biscuits
Milk

Hot beef and vegetables
Buttered bread
Apple muffins
Milk

Creamed chicken with carrots
   and potatoes
Buttered rolls
Unsweetened fruit juice

Macaroni and cheese
Tomato and lettuce salad
Buttered rolls
Mandarin or plain orange
Milk

Egg salad sandwich, with lettuce
Cream of tomato soup
Canned unsweetened fruit
Cookies
Milk

Cream of carrot soup
Salmon salad on lettuce
Buttered hot dog roll
Banana
Milk

Cream of chicken soup
Bread sticks
Wedge of cheese
Cherry tomatoes
Cold baked apple
Milk

Ham sandwich
Vegetable salad
Peanut butter cookies
Milk

Cream of tomato soup
Potato and celery salad
Cold ham and Melba toast
Grapes
Milk

Cream of mushroom soup
Bread sticks
Ham sandwich with lettuce
Orange
Milk

Hot Swiss steak with vegetables
Buttered bread
Applesauce
Milk

Note: The amount of each ingredient varies according to the exchanges of your own diet. As a substitute for milk, or if you can't afford the exchange, use low-calorie diet drinks as a beverage.

LUNCHES FOR WORK

For calculating the exchange values of sandwiches for packed lunches, you should memorize a few of the exchanges and experiment with their various substitutes.

— A commercial slice of bread — white, whole, or cracked wheat = **one** Bread Exchange.
— 2 slices of sandwich bread (i.e., thinly sliced), with crusts removed, are equal to **one** Bread Exchange.
— 1, 2" diameter dinner roll = 1 Bread Exchange.
— 1 hamburger or hot dog roll = 2 Bread Eychanges.

Some samples below will illustrate the various ways in which you can switch exchanges.

Example 1

If your diet indicates the following number of exchanges for your meal:

> 2 Bread Exchanges
> 3 Meat Exchanges
> 2 Fat Exchanges

Here's what you can do with those exchanges, according to your own preferences.

A. For one sandwich, made with 2 slices of regular bread:
The filling can include

> 2 teaspoons butter and 3 oz lean meat
> **or** 2 teaspoons butter and 3 hard-boiled eggs
> **or** 3 oz canned meat or pâté
> **or** 3 oz Cheddar cheese (3 slices)
> **or** 2 teaspoons butter and 3 oz canned fish, well drained
> **or** 2 teaspoons butter and 2 oz cold meat, plus a hard-boiled egg
> **or** 2 teaspoons butter, 2 oz cold meat, and 1 slice of Cheddar cheese

B. For 2 sandwiches, made with 4 slices of thin sandwich bread, crusts removed.
The filling can include half of any of the amounts listed above.
Example: 1 teaspoon butter and 1 ½ oz cold meat.

C. For 3 sandwiches made with 6 slices of thin sandwich bread, crusts removed.

The filling can include any of the amounts listed above, divided by 3.

Example: butter 6 slices of bread with 2 teaspoons butter, and fill each sandwich with 1 oz meat, 1 egg, or 1 oz of Cheddar cheese.

D. 1 hamburger = 3 oz meat, garnished with mustard, catsup, and a slice of tomato.

or 1 hot dog, plus 2 oz of cheese

or 2 hot dogs (but only 1 bun), plus 1 oz cheese, **or** 1 egg

or 1 smoked meat, made with 3 oz lean meat

= 1 Bread Exchange (4″ x 3″ thin rye bread is usually used)
3 Meat Exchanges
1 Fat Exchange

Example 2

If the number of exchanges per meal is as follows:

1 Bread Exchange
2 Meat Exchanges
1 Fat Exchange

Then you can make these substitutes:

A. For 1 sandwich made with 2 slices of thin sandwich bread, crusts removed:

1 teaspoon butter and 2 oz lean meat

or 1 teaspoon butter and 2 eggs

or 2 oz canned meat or pâté

or 2 oz Cheddar cheese

or 1 teaspoon butter, 1 oz meat, and 1 egg

or 2 tablespoons peanut butter

or 1 teaspoon butter, 1 oz cheese, and 1 egg

or 1 teaspoon butter, 1 oz cheese, and 1 oz meat

B. For 1 sandwich, made with 2 slices of ordinary bread, omit the vegetable exchanges for this meal, and use the same amount of fillings as in Example A above.

C. For 2 sandwiches, made with 4 slices of thin sandwich bread, crusts removed, omit the vegetable exchanges for this meal, and use half the amounts indicated in Example A.
Example: use 1 teaspoon butter for all the bread, and fill with 1 oz cold meat, or 1 egg, or 1 slice cheese.

Other fillings:

— Cottage cheese, beaten smooth, with a banana or strawberries (the fruit exchange), and lemon juice.
— Eggs scrambled without butter or oil, and broiled mushrooms (the vegetable exchange)
— Chopped frankfurters, hard-boiled egg, and Chili sauce.
— Minced veal with chopped green pepper and cabbage (the vegetable exchange).

D. 1 hamburger made with 2 oz meat (omit the vegetable exchange for this meal)
or 1 hot dog and either 1 oz cheese, or 1 egg (omit vegetable exchange)
or 1 smoked Meat sandwich, made with 2 oz lean meat
Note: In A, B, and D in Examples 1 and 2, the required vegetable, fruit, or milk exchanges have been left out.
In the case of D above, when eating in a restaurant, subtract the fat exchanges if the bread or rolls are served buttered. If you are given too much or too little meat, bread, or butter, simply redistribute the amounts into the proportions given in our examples.
Remember also that lettuce, chopped celery, dill, unsweetened relish, mustard, mayonnaise (special), and all the seasonings can help improve the appearance and taste of sandwiches.

Other suggestions for sandwich fillings:

— Chopped hard-boiled egg with chopped cold beets (subtract Vegetable Exchange).
— Chicken, chopped celery, and curry powder.
— Chopped ham and unsweetened relish.
— Chopped sausage, cream cheese (subtract Fat Exchange), and 1 teaspoon minced onion.
— Cream cheese (subtract Fat Exchange) and raisins (subtract Fruit Exchange).

— Creamed cottage cheese with raisins.
— Creamed cottage cheese with crisp bacon
— Scrambled eggs (use no fat), and chopped ham
— Scrambled eggs (no fat), and crisp bacon
— Scrambled eggs (no fat) and Cheddar cheese, with Worcestershire sauce
— Sardines and cucumber (vegetable exchange)
— Canned salmon and cucumber.

Some Exchanges to Remember

No matter what sort of meal you plan to prepare, the exchanges below are useful ones to memorize:

1. Fruit Exchanges

1 Fruit Exchange can be replaced by:

1 portion unsweetened fruit juice	orange	3½	oz
	grapefruit	3½	oz
	apple	3	oz
	pineapple	3	oz
	prune	2	oz
	grape	2	oz
1 portion vegetable juice	V8 (or other)	8	oz
1 tomato juice		8	oz
1 fruit mashed or blended into other ingredients			

2. Bread Exchanges

1 Bread Exchange can be replaced by:

1 portion cooked cereal (made with water)	cooked oatmeal	½ cup
	cooked cream of wheat	½ cup
1 portion pasta	cooked rice	⅓ cup
	other pasta, cooked	⅓ cup
1 helping dessert	regular jello	3½ oz (2½" cube)
	stewed fruit, no sugar	¾ cup
1 beverage	ginger ale	6 oz
	Coke or Pepsi	4 oz
1 fruit juice	orange juice or grapefruit juice	5½ oz

	apple juice or	
	pineapple juice	4½ oz
	prune or grape juice	3 oz
1 vegetable	mashed potato	½ cup
	creamed corn	½ cup
	mashed parsnip	½ cup
1 yogurt	vanilla. coffee, or	
	plain	5 oz

3. Meat Exchanges

Equivalent to the same amount of meat ground or chopped and used in stock, soup, Oxo, Bovril, or consommé.
1 beaten egg or 2 egg whites (add 1 fat exchange).

4. Vegetable Exchanges

Same as for fruits, as well as any puréed vegetable used in bouillon or soup.

5. Fat Exchanges

1 oz cream (in drinks or on fruit)
1 exchange of butter, melted (for bouillon, soup, or vegetable purées)
1 oz oil (for bouillon, or vegetable purées)
1 slice lean, crisp bacon, whole or crumbled
1 tablespoon whipping cream
1 tablespoon commercial vinaigrette dressing
1 tablespoon cream cheese, with relish, chive, or green pepper added
5 small stuffed olives

6. Partial or Mixed Exchanges

Postum: made with 2 tablespoons Postum and water = ½ Bread Exchange
Soups: for exchanges, refer to the commercial brands listed in the chapters on Soups; 1 portion = 3⅓ oz of a 10-oz can, before diluting with water, or 7 oz diluted.
Juice and milk: 4 oz skim milk and 1 fruit juice = 1 Bread Exchange.
1 oz meat and 1 Group B Vegetable Exchange = 1 Bread Exchange.

All the light meals listed in the Snack section that follows are
equivalent to:
— 1 Bread Exchange + 1 Meat Exchange + 1 Group B
Vegetable Exchange + 1 Fat Exchange.
— 1 Bread Exchange + 1 Meat Exchange + 1 Fruit Exchange
+ 1 Fat Exchange.
— 2 Bread Exchanges + ½ Meat Exchange + 1½ Fat
Exchanges.

Evening Snacks

These snacks have the same approximate value (to within one unit)
as the "light meal" most diets permit — 8 oz milk and 1 Bread
Exchange. These substitutions can also be used at any meal.

1
8 oz milk
¾ cup cornflakes

2
8 oz milk
3 Graham crackers

3
8 oz skim milk
⅔ cup ice cream

4
8 oz skim milk
20 large potato chips

5
Black tea or coffee
1 slice bread
2 tablespoons peanut butter
1 portion fresh fruit

6
8 oz tomato juice
1 oz Cheddar cheese
6, 2" sq. soda crackers

7
8 oz tomato juice

8
6 oz plain yogurt

6 Melba toasts
3 sardines
6 small olives

4 small dry cookies
coffee, 1 oz 15% cream

9
3½ oz orange juice
2 slices bread (no crusts)
1 scrambled egg
1 teaspoon butter
lettuce and mustard

10
8 oz V8
7 Ritz crackers
5 medium shrimp
½ tablespoon mayonnaise

11
8 oz tomato juice
2 slices bread (crusts removed)
1 thin slice lean ham (1 oz)
1 teaspoon butter
lettuce and mustard

12
Black tea or coffee
2 slices bread (crusts removed)
3 slices lean, crisp bacon
1 tomato
Lettuce, and Zero Mayonnaise
½ portion fruit, no sugar

13
Black tea or coffee
1 whole slice bread
   (or 2 without crusts)
1 oz cold meat
1 teaspoon butter
Lettuce
1 portion fresh fruit

14
Black tea or coffee
2 oz or 4 tablespoons 15% cream
4 tablespoons cottage cheese
6 pieces Melba toast
⅓ cup pineapple, no sugar

15
Black tea or coffee
1½ oz steak
Green Salad
1 tablespoon vinaigrette
   dressing

16
Green salad
1 hard-boiled egg, or 5 shrimp
½ tablespoon mayonnaise
1½ rusks, or
1, ½" thick slice French bread

½ cup peas, or ⅔ cup carrots	Black tea or coffee
1 portion fruit, no sugar	½ portion fruit, no sugar

17

4 oz pineapple juice,
   unsweetened
7 Ritz crackers
1½ wedges Gruyère cheese,
   or 1 oz Cheddar

18

Black tea or coffee
2 slices bread
1 egg, hard-boiled or fried in
   butter
1 teaspoon butter
Lettuce, and Zero Mayonnaise

19

Eggnogg (good for a liquid diet):
whip together
4 oz milk
1 egg
1, 6″ banana

20

Milkshake
whip together
8 oz milk
1, 5″ banana
flavoring

21

Soup:
⅓ cup cooked rice (exactly
   measured)
1 oz chopped chicken
chicken stock (optional)
4 soda crackers
1 teaspoon butter

22

Black coffee or tea
⅔ cup cooked spaghetti (exactly)
1 oz meatballs
½ cup spaghetti sauce (see chapter on sauces) — no value
1 teaspoon butter

Practical Suggestions

1. Vary salads by using watercress, escarole, red cabbage, chinese cabbage, endive, romaine, and fresh spinach.

2. Several casserole recipes can be frozen in individual portions, and used later, one at a time, so that you don't have to eat the same thing several days in a row.

3. Baked potatoes can be cooked in thick aluminum foil, frozen, and then reheated in the same wrapping.

4. For people who eat at home, it's easier to measure a daily portion of milk and keep it separate from the supply used by the rest of the family; take what you need from this special container as needed.

5. Buttermilk biscuits: keep the dough, in 6- or 10-biscuit packages, in the refrigerator, ready to be cooked and used in a number of ways:
   — as a Bread Exchange substitute (1 roll = 1 Exchange).
   — add cheese or crisp bacon before baking (½ Meat Exchange per 1 Bread Exchange).
   — rolled lightly before baking, it can be used as shortcake.
   — serve a 3″ square piece of shortcake covered with an exchange of fruit, and topped with special whipped cream (see chapter on Desserts).
   — make cinnamon rolls by rolling out the dough and sprinkling with cinnamon and powdered sugar substitute.

6. An easy way to reheat any kind of roll: sprinkle them with a spoonful of water, place in a brown paper bag, and warm in a slow oven.

7. Potatoes put through a ricer can be cooked in quantity, and frozen in an airtight container. They can easily be used any time; reheat them by steaming or using them in a croquette recipe or other dish.

8. Many of the new saucepans and frying pans let you cook without using any fat. A visit to the household appliance section of any large department store will show you what is available to meet your own needs; the choice is becoming bigger and better.

9. Onions, like mushrooms, should be sautéed slowly in a thick frying pan, over gentle heat. They can be prepared ahead of time and kept a day or two in the refrigerator. All you have to do as they cook is add a few drops of water or stock to keep them from sticking, and to assure a good brown color.

10. Try the same technique using very thin slices of raw potatoes. They demand a bit more attention to keep them browning evenly, but you'll end up with golden fried potatoes, without having to use butter. Measure the potatoes before slicing; it looks like much more after cooking.

11. For holidays or special occasions, don't hesitate to use all the possibilities suggested for food with little or no exchange value — for at least the illusion of a real banquet.

12. For days when you don't feel like eating much, make a list of recipes that include a number of meal exchanges in one small dish. A one-dish meal is easier to take than several courses.

13. Check the "sweetening power" of the sugar substitute you use. This value varies from product to product, and is indicated on the container. Use less rather than more; it's easier to add a few drops than to waste a whole recipe.

14. Take a good look at any product labelled "dietetic"; they can be useless to you, or even harmful. Check their ingredients closely — they ought to be clearly listed if they are intended for calculated diets. Don't forget that some of these products are meant for other types of diets, such as salt-restricted or low animal-fat diets. Some products, even though they are low-calorie, are still part of the exchange system, and can be used only in certain amounts. If you are ever in any doubt about using a certain product, consult your doctor or dietician for the answer. Some commercial diet drinks can be a welcome change of pace or supplement to your menu, and the number of interesting new products is growing.

15. It's easier to determine portions if you buy wrapped meat marked with the exact weight. Portions can be frozen individually.
Example: if you buy 16 oz of lean minced meat, and your exchange is 3 oz, divide the package into 4 equal parts (4 oz each); after cooking these will give 3-oz portions.